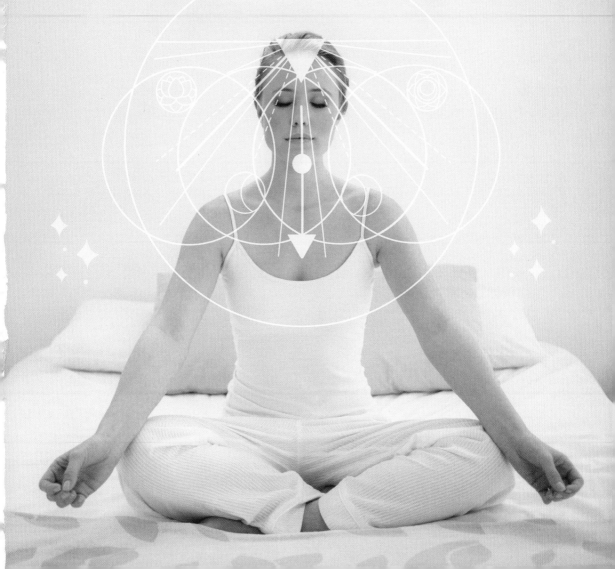

BREATHWORK
for
Self-transformation

BREATHWORK

for

Self-transformation

Harness
your vital energy for
health and happiness

KONSTANTINOS TSELIOS

SIRIUS

SIRIUS

This edition published in 2024 by Sirius Publishing, a division of
Arcturus Publishing Limited,
26/27 Bickels Yard, 151–153 Bermondsey Street,
London SE1 3HA

All images courtesy of Shutterstock

ISBN: 978-1-3988-3669-3
AD010765UK
Designer: Sally Bond

Printed in China

Contents

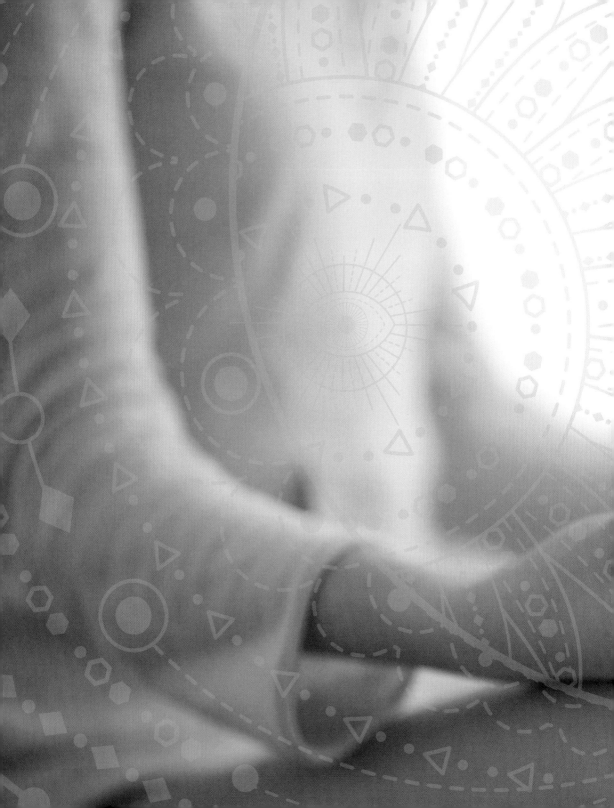

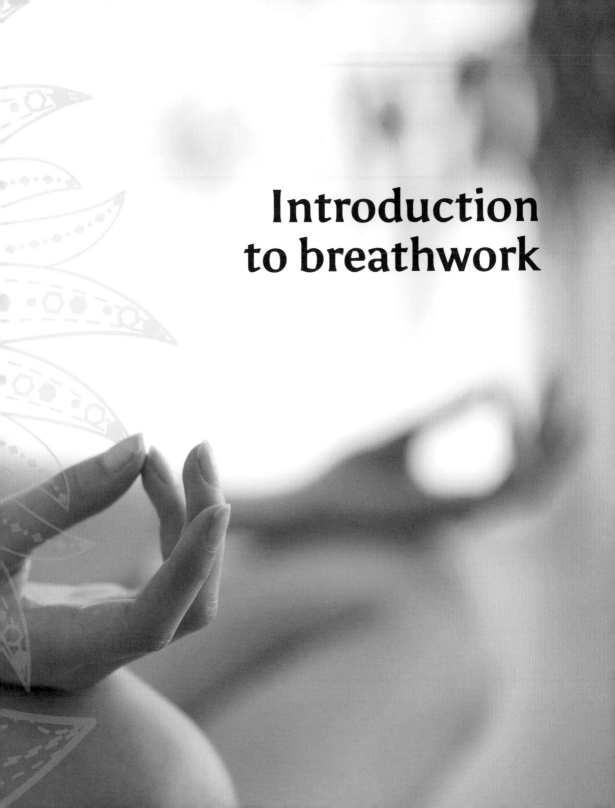

Introduction
to breathwork

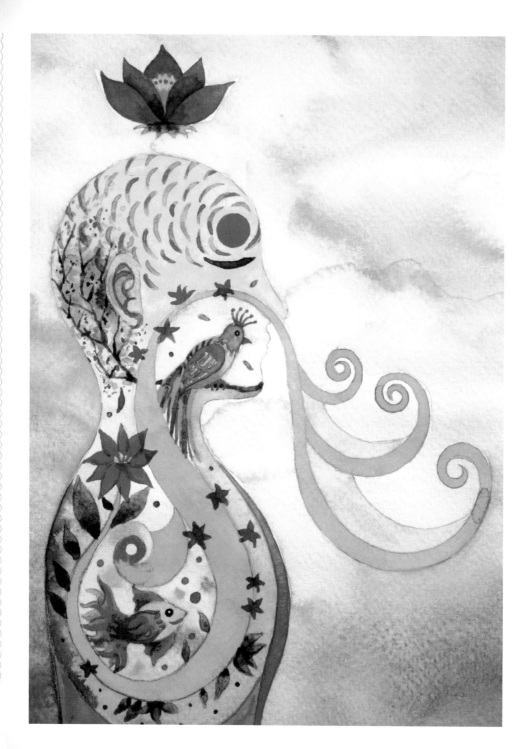

Most of us are now well aware of the benefits of a good, healthy diet and also of the importance of regular exercise. There's also a big commercial interest in promoting healthy eating and exercise, with everyone from food companies to fitness machine manufacturers making a lot of money and then spending much of it on advertising and promotion to further spread the message.

However, there's one area of healthy living which gets largely ignored, perhaps partly because there's no money to be made. It relies on a resource that's all around us, is totally free for everyone to use, and is simply referred to as 'air'. As the 1960s British pop band The Hollies sang in their famous hit, 'All I need is the air that I breathe…'

Our basic necessities for survival are oxygen, water and food and, in terms of importance these could be ranked from oxygen as the most important to food as the least important. We can survive days without food, hours without water but only minutes without the air that we breathe.

With that in mind, it's amazing how little we think about the importance of breathing and the air that surrounds us. Our body breathes automatically without us even thinking about it, plus the air is always there, so why give it a thought?

Tuning your engine

If you speak to anyone in the motor industry who tunes engines to make them run faster and more efficiently, they will tell you that three of the main areas they concentrate on are the intake of fuel, the intake of air and the removal of waste gases. Mechanics will even go as far as polishing some of the metal surfaces within an engine so that the air flows more efficiently into the combustion chamber and the burned gases flow more efficiently out of the engine. Done properly this can make the engine both more powerful and also more efficient on fuel.

We can look at the human body in a similar way when it comes to breathing. The way that we take in air and exhale it can make a big difference to the efficiency and wellbeing of our bodies and also to our minds.

This is something that has been recognized for thousands of years, with the ancient Vedic and Ayurvedic texts in India referring to the importance of breathing techniques when it comes to improving health as well as directly treating some health problems. In addition, breathing techniques play an important part in the practice of yoga, to keep the body fully supplied with oxygen while yoga postures or 'asanas' are being practiced.

There are also yogic breathing techniques which are used on their own and not as part of an asana. These techniques are sometimes used to maximize the oxygen in the body as part of a yoga session, providing a sort of 'oxygen buzz' which can make some people feel a little dizzy to start with. Done properly, though, it can be a very mind-focusing and inspiring part of a yoga session.

The use of different breathing techniques is also important when it comes to meditation. The concentration on breathing is often used at the start of meditation practice, to help focus the mind and stop it from being distracted. It has even been said that controlling the breath is so important that it is an essential starting point for understanding the mind and the body.

My own experience

As a yoga and mindfulness teacher myself, I am well aware of the importance of breathing techniques, both when it comes to yoga asanas and also during meditation. One of my old yoga gurus in India once told me that the practice of yoga should ideally consist of 20% yoga asanas (postures), 30% breathing and 50% meditation.

To him, breathing was a more important part of yoga practice than the yoga asanas or postures, which many people think of as the main component of yoga. Meditation forms an even more important part of proper yoga practice and this also relies to an extent on breathing techniques. When I am teaching meditation, or just meditating on my own, I often start by concentrating on breathing, which helps to clear the mind of other distractions and then leads into full meditation.

Boost your own health and wellbeing

In this book, I have set out to explain some of the fundamentals of breathing and breathwork, including a scientific look at the workings of the human body when it comes to the intake, use and exhalation of air.

I also want to give you some breathing exercises that you can use every day to help boost your health and wellbeing. You can easily fit breathing exercises into your daily life, perhaps during a lunch hour or when you get home from work. You may find that some simple breathing exercises will help to reduce stress, which could be a real bonus if you work in a stressful environment.

Reducing stress and focusing your mind with breathing techniques should also help with your mental health and wellbeing, which in turn will help with your physical health.

In modern society, scientists and medics are slowly realizing the importance of the mind when it comes to physical health as well as mental health. However, this link between mind, body and also spirit is something that the ancients were talking about thousands of years ago, particularly in the Indian Vedic texts which even pre-date most current religions. In some ways, we are now going back to the future, to recapture some old techniques and ways of thinking that can help us survive better in the modern day.

I hope this book will give you some inspiration to begin your own regular breathing exercises and perhaps even encourage you to take up yoga or start practising meditation.

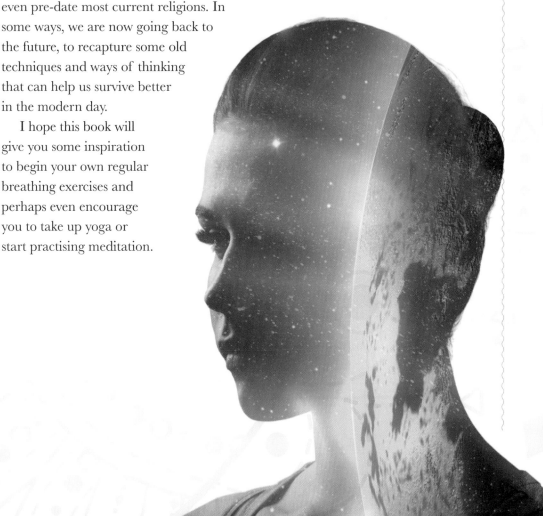

THE BIOLOGY OF BREATHING

Kicking off with a bit of a science lesson is the best way to illustrate the mechanics of breathing and how it affects all parts of the body.

Starting at the smallest, cellular level, every cell in our bodies needs a constant supply of food and nutrients as well as water and oxygen. Each cell powers itself by combining the food or 'fuel' with the oxygen and 'burning' this mixture to create the energy for life. Each cell can be seen as a tiny motorcar engine, burning fuel with oxygen to power itself.

Of course, this 'burning' process is actually a chemical reaction that is very slow at cellular level, so there are no flames or fire, just a continuous generation of energy. This 'burning' is technically referred to as oxidation, where the calories in food are combined with oxygen and are oxidized to create energy.

In a motorcar engine the 'food' is petrol and this is a very volatile liquid so it oxidizes with an explosion. In the cells of our bodies, the food is usually some form of carbohydrate and this 'burns' or oxidizes with oxygen at a slow rate, creating energy and heat as well as the waste product of carbon dioxide.

This 'burning' process takes place within specific parts of each cell called mitochondria. These contain enzymes that drive the process and then transfer the

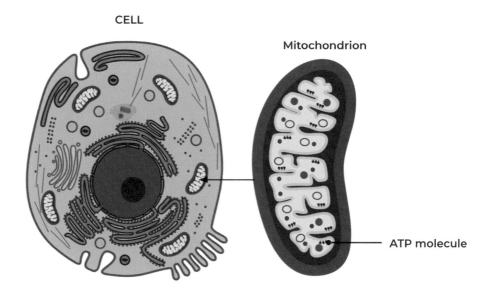

CELL

Mitochondrion

ATP molecule

energy released into a storage molecule called adenosine triphosphate or ATP. This is the basic store of energy seen in most living things and could be likened to a small battery pack which keeps cells alive.

This energy generation at cellular level is the most important part of human metabolism and it also generates the body heat that we need as warm-blooded mammals. It's one of the reasons that our bodies can burn as many as 2,000 calories each day, even if we don't do much exercise

Supplying the cells

So, the actual process and chemical reaction of respiration takes place at a cellular level within our bodies, where the fuel of food is 'burned' with oxygen to create the energy for life.

The systems we normally think of within our bodies, such as the nose, windpipe and lungs are just part of the supply system needed to get the oxygen to the individual cells. The heart and the circulatory system are also needed to send this oxygen to the individual cells via the bloodstream and to remove the waste products such as carbon dioxide.

The breathing process starts when our chest muscles, including the large muscle membrane under our lungs called the diaphragm, pull down and causes air to be sucked in through our nose and down to our lungs.

Being nosy

Ironically, the one thing most of us are never nosy enough to want to know more about is our own nose! Apart from perhaps being worried about its cosmetic shape or size, most of us don't think about what our nose is actually there for.

As part of the respiratory system, the nose is actually a deliberate bottleneck. It's much quicker to breathe large amounts of air in through our mouths, bypassing the nose, and we often do this when we are out of breath, perhaps after a run or other sporting activity.

So, why do we need a nose, then, why not just use our mouths all the time? Well, the nose does much more than just take in air, it also acts as a filter, with nose hairs and mucus taking out some of the dust and impurities in the air. It also helps to

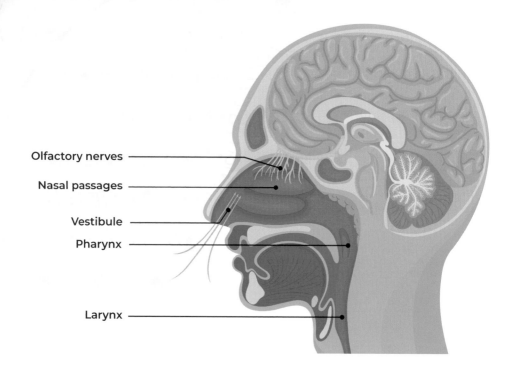

Olfactory nerves

Nasal passages

Vestibule

Pharynx

Larynx

warm the incoming air as well as moisturizing it. (If you've ever spent a long time in a dry, air-conditioned room you'll appreciate how hard this can be on your airways.)

If you want to test the importance of nasal breathing, just close your nose for a few minutes and breathe only through your mouth. You'll soon start to feel that your throat is feeling dry and you may even start coughing. For this reason, nearly all breathwork exercises involve inhaling through the nose only, though some may require you to exhale through the mouth.

With many different functions and tasks to undertake, including the production of mucus, the human nose has also adapted itself to suit specific environments. So, for instance, people whose ancestors originated in cold or dry climates have often evolved longer, thinner noses so that the air they breathe can be processed before it hits the lungs, making it warmer and moister. Those whose ancestors originate in warm, moist environments, such as tropical jungles, can have shorter noses with more open nostrils.

Once air has flowed through the external part of the nose, it reaches the nasal cavity, which sits above the mouth cavity and below the cavities in the top of our head which hold our brain and eyes. Air then feeds into the top of the mouth cavity before heading down the windpipe to our lungs.

Everything is very close and connected in our heads and there are even internal tubes called eustachian tubes which connect our inner ears to our mouth cavity and are designed to keep the inner ears at an atmospheric air pressure.

This series of interconnections also leads to vulnerability and is why a nose infection can often spread to a throat, lung or ear infection. When you consider that the nasal cavity is just under the brain, you can see how infections here can also lead to headaches.

The mucus produced in the nose plays an important part in stopping infections by capturing and killing bugs and microbes as well as cleaning the nasal cavity. The mucus is produced by the mucous membrane which covers the sides of the nasal cavity and this membrane contains millions of small hair-like structures called *cilia*. These keep the mucus in continual movement, with waste mucus eventually entering our throats and leaving through our digestive system.

For a healthy nasal system, the mucus needs to be of the correct consistency and moisture. If it is too dried out, then microbes can bed in and cause an infection such as a cold, which in turn can lead to very watery mucus as the body tries to fight the infection. It is even thought that some foods can affect the consistency of mucus, with dairy products in particular thought to create thicker mucus.

Even our tears find their way into our nasal cavity, since there's a tiny duct at the bottom of each eye cavity which feeds the excess salty water that lubricates our eyes down into the top of the nasal cavity where it drains away. This is why our noses will often begin to run during weeping, when an excess of tears starts to water down the mucus in our nasal cavity.

The other important function of the nose, of course, is our sense of smell and this is taken care of by the olfactory nerve at the top of the nasal cavity. It has nerve endings here which are responsible for the sense of smell. When we have colds or flu, the excess build-up of mucus can cover these nerve endings, thus reducing our sense of smell.

Honeymoon nose

There's another, quite surprising feature of the nose that is really only talked about by doctors and specialists in ear, nose and throat medicine. Under the mucous membrane there's a layer of erectile tissue which works in a similar way to the erectile tissue in the penis and clitoris.

This tissue contains small passageways which can become engorged with blood, causing them to expand and become harder.

There's a connection between all the areas in the body that contain this erectile tissue which has led to doctors diagnosing a condition called 'honeymoon nose.' This is where one or both members of a couple who have been very sexually active can find that the lining of their nose becomes expanded and this starts to block the nose a little.

Research into this phenomenon over the years has even suggested a link between menstrual cramps in women and the inflammation of some areas of the lining of the nose. It was found that if these areas of inflammation were treated with a gentle anesthetic then the menstrual pain would go away. This even led to a severe type of experimental treatment where some of the nerve endings in the nose were destroyed with cauterization to try and reduce menstrual pain, though this is obviously no longer practised.

Alternating nostrils

Research into the linings of the nose has shown that the expansion of this erectile tissue in the nose lining usually takes place on an alternating basis. So, while the tissue in one nostril is expanded, reducing the space for airflow, the tissue in the neighboring nostril stays at its normal level and does not expand.

This alternation takes place on a continual basis so, at any one time, most of us are using one nostril more than the other, with a change-over then happening naturally after an hour or two. This can be seen as part of a continual maintenance process in the nose, where one nostril is given time to recover and have more blood flow, while the other is doing most of the work.

This alternation of nostrils is something that was recognized thousands of years ago and working for short periods to control which nostril is being used the most

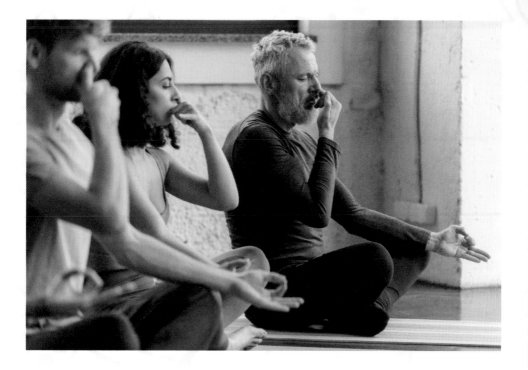

forms part of yogic breathing practice, with the main technique being alternate-nasal breathing, or Nadi Shodhanam. I will detail this exercise later in the book, as one of the many simple breathing exercises which are easy to undertake.

This natural process of alternation between the nostrils is technically known as an 'infradian rhythm' and modern research is starting to indicate what many yogis have known for years – that each nostril can have an effect on different parts of our body and mind. In the same way that we sometimes talk about 'left-brain thinking' or 'right-brain thinking', with some people being more driven by one side of their brain and the type of thinking that goes with this, then predominant use of a particular nostril may also have wider effects.

For instance, in some types of yoga it is thought that if people tend to breathe more through their right nostril they are more active and even more aggressive, as well as being more focused on the material world. Those who breathe predominantly through their left nostril are said to be more passive and quiet, focusing more on their internal world.

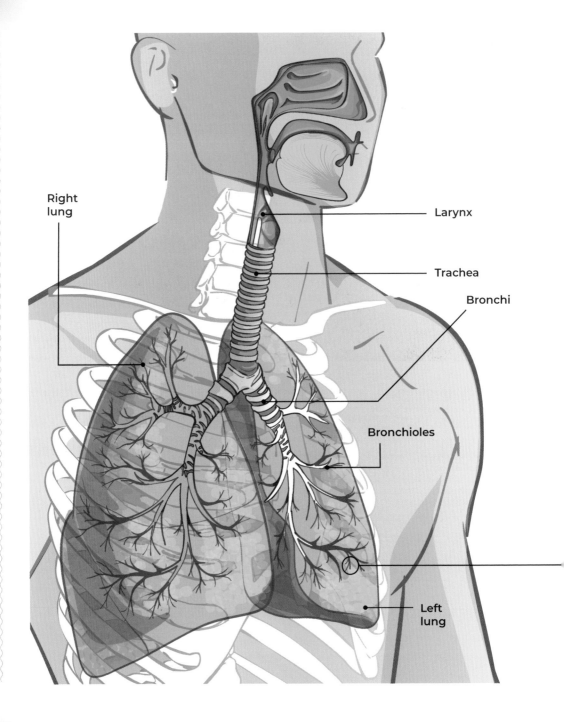

Right
lung

Larynx

Trachea

Bronchi

Bronchioles

Left
lung

Some types of yoga, such as svara yoga, even correlated each nostril to the workings of particular internal organs and processes such as digestion. Students of this type of yoga would open their right nostril before eating as this was thought to stimulate digestion. Drinking was seen as a more passive process so was undertaken with the left nostril more open.

Into the lungs

Of course, there's much more to breathing than just the nose and an equally important consideration when it comes to breathwork is how the lungs work. A lot of breathwork for health is based around how we fill our lungs, what rhythm we use when filling them and what part of our chest we concentrate on when breathing.

It's worth having a quick look at the mechanics of the lungs, to see how they work and how we can work with them to improve their efficiency.

Once air has passed through our nose, it passes through our throat in a passageway which is shared with our food or liquid called the pharynx, before it reaches the larynx which is also called the voice box.

The larynx has a flap of cartilage at its top, called the epiglottis, which folds forward when we swallow, closing off the larynx so that food doesn't go into our lungs. When we drink or eat, sometimes things 'go down the wrong way' when the epiglottis has not closed properly and food or liquid heads into the larynx, causing us to cough or choke.

Just below the larynx is the trachea or windpipe, which splits into two to allow air to enter both sides of the lungs. Once inside the lungs, the air enters ever-smaller passageways called bronchioles and ends up at small sacs called alveoli, which under a microscope can look like a bunch of grapes.

Alveoli

The process of exchange of air takes place in the membrane walls of the small alveoli, called the respiratory membrane. Here, the oxygen in the air is passed through into the bloodstream and the waste carbon dioxide gas from the blood is passed back into the lungs and then breathed out.

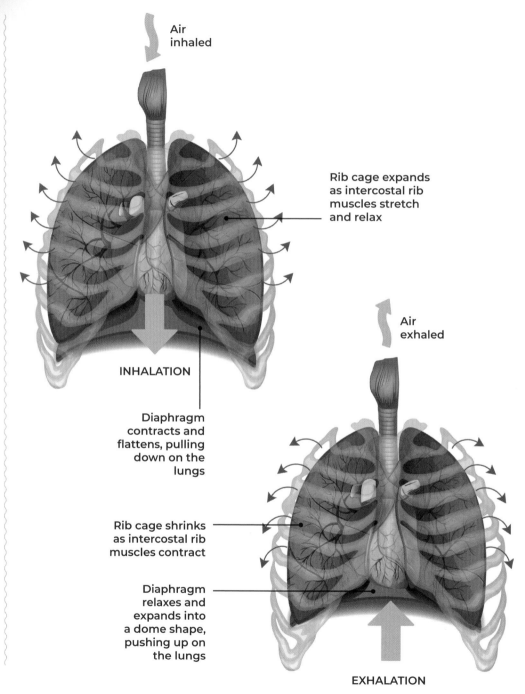

Air
inhaled

Rib cage expands
as intercostal rib
muscles stretch
and relax

INHALATION

Diaphragm
contracts and
flattens, pulling
down on the
lungs

Air
exhaled

Rib cage shrinks
as intercostal rib
muscles contract

Diaphragm
relaxes and
expands into
a dome shape,
pushing up on
the lungs

EXHALATION

The muscles behind breathing

Although they do all the work of transferring oxygen into the blood and removing carbon dioxide, the lungs themselves do not contain the muscles that drive their own operation. Instead, this work is done by the diaphragm, a dome-shape sheet of muscle that sits under the lungs in the chest cavity, as well as by the intercostal muscles between each of the ribs, plus the clavicle or collarbone muscles.

When the intercostal muscles expand, they pull the ribs apart and increase the size of the chest cavity, causing the lungs to suck in air to fill the vacuum. When they contract, the chest cavity shrinks and air is expelled from the lungs. Most of us use this type of chest breathing when we are in a relaxed state, with just shallow breaths since our body does not need so much oxygen when it is relaxed.

When the collarbone muscles expand and raise the collarbone they also increase the size of the chest cavity and cause the intake of air. However, this type of breathing is usually only needed when we are really out of breath, perhaps after sporting activity. You might have seen runners after a race when their shoulders are going up and down as they try to inhale as much air as possible.

The only muscle that's specifically used for breathing is the large diaphragm muscle. When this muscle contracts and becomes flatter, it pulls down on the lungs above, causing them open and suck in air, so that we breathe in. When the diaphragm muscle then relaxes, it goes back to its domed shape and pushes up, forcing out the air in the lungs so that we breathe out.

The diaphragm works in conjunction with the other muscles, with all three types of breathing used when we are very short of breath, after intensive physical activity.

In breathwork exercises the two main types of breathing referred to when it comes to sucking air into the lungs are 'diaphragm or diaphragmatic breathing,' where we concentrate on using the diaphragm to pull in air, as well as 'chest breathing,' where we concentrate our minds on expanding and raising the intercostal muscles. A third type of breathing, using just our collarbone or clavicle muscles to pull in air is rarely practised on its own during breathwork, but these muscles may naturally be working when we are doing chest or diaphragmatic breathing.

When we are inactive, we typically take around 15 breaths per minute but this can more than double during hard exercise. The rate of breathing is automatically controlled by the respiratory centre in the brain stem, but you can deliberately alter your breathing rate if you want and this ability to change our breathing rhythm when we want is an important part of many breathing exercises.

It's in the blood

The final step in getting oxygen to the cells that need it is the bloodstream. Our hearts pump blood all round our bodies and, when it passes the respiratory membranes in the lungs, an exchange of gases takes place with oxygen taken into the blood and carbon dioxide removed from it.

While some gases can be contained in the saline liquid of the blood itself, most of the oxygen in the blood is transported in the hemoglobin molecule which is found in red blood cells. This molecule has four protein chains attached to an atom of iron and it is this atom of iron that attracts and holds the oxygen gas and transports it via the red blood cells in the bloodstream. It is this oxygen and iron combination that gives the red blood cells and therefore the whole bloodstream its red colouration. The hemoglobin can also carry carbon dioxide, which it picks up from the cells and returns to the lungs in the bloodstream.

Hemoglobin also has an affinity for other gases, notably the carbon monoxide that is found in cigarette smoke or exhaust fumes from cars or domestic boilers. Hemoglobin has an attraction for carbon monoxide that is 240 times more than that for oxygen so, when breathed in, carbon monoxide quickly fills up most of the space in the red blood cells that should be reserved for oxygen thus causing the cells in the body to be starved of oxygen, which can in extreme cases lead to death.

Apparently people who smoke can have up to 15% of their hemoglobin fixed with carbon monoxide, and effectively useless, even if they are not actively smoking at that particular moment.

When the blood flows through the tiny blood vessels that run next to individual cells in our body, a process occurs which is similar to that in the respiratory membrane in the lungs, with oxygen passing into the cells and carbon dioxide being expelled back into the bloodstream.

OXYGEN AND HEMOGLOBIN

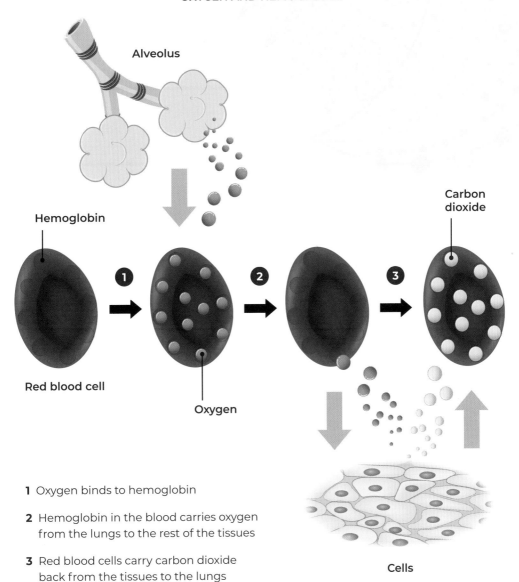

Alveolus

Hemoglobin

Carbon
dioxide

Red blood cell

Oxygen

Cells

1 Oxygen binds to hemoglobin

2 Hemoglobin in the blood carries oxygen
from the lungs to the rest of the tissues

3 Red blood cells carry carbon dioxide
back from the tissues to the lungs

USING BREATHWORK TO BOOST YOUR ENERGY LEVELS

Having looked at the biology of breathing, you can see how this is the essential generator of energy in our bodies, equally as important as the food we take in. While many of us spend time worrying about a healthy diet, how many of us worry about our breathing, about the strength of our respiratory system and the quality of the air we are breathing in?

As I mentioned earlier, the respiration process at cellular level combines oxygen with the fuel of food, to create the energy we need for life. This is then stored in the mitochondria within each cell which are like mini battery packs that power our bodies.

So, when we undertake breathwork it's a bit like putting an electric car on fast charge, to quickly boost its energy levels. Most of us just carry out our daily lives without thinking about our breathing and this could be likened to charging an electric car on slow charge.

If you add some regular breathwork exercise into your daily routine, you'll boost your energy levels and this can have a direct effect on both your physical and mental health.

Most of us breathe by using our chest muscles rather than using the full force of our diaphragm muscle. We take small, shallow breaths rather than large, deep ones. This tends to mean that the air we breathe in stays near the top of the lungs.

Due to the force of gravity, much of the blood that flows past the membranes in our lungs is at a lower level. So, when we take shallow breaths, just using our chest muscles, we're not getting as much air to the most efficient part of the lungs, where there is plenty of blood ready to capture the oxygen in the air.

By undertaking breathwork that involves increased diaphragm breathing we can oxygenate our blood much more efficiently and the increased suction pressure of the diaphragm muscle is also thought to help the heart by pushing some of the returning blood back via the heart and into our lungs.

This type of diaphragmatic breathing is a fundamental part of breathwork and it is simple to learn. However, you have to spend time consciously cultivating it before it becomes an automatic process. Having said that, even if you just put a

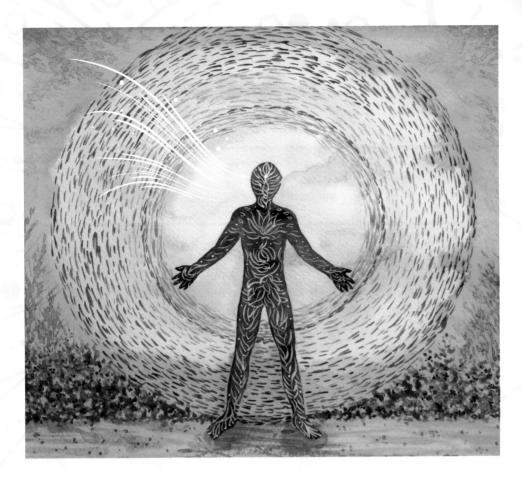

few minutes aside each day to practice diaphragmatic breathing, or other types of breathwork, you will still feel the benefits in terms of extra energy and vitality.

You might think it's strange to have to learn to breathe properly in this way, since surely our bodies will do that automatically. Well, just think about an infant learning to walk. If it wasn't encouraged and trained to walk by its parents, an infant might spend its entire life crawling on all fours. It's only by training and hard work that an infant turns walking into an automatic process. The same can be said with breathwork. It might take some training but if you concentrate on proper, deep diaphragmic breathing during breathwork exercises, it will eventually become as natural as walking.

THE BENEFITS OF REGULAR BREATHWORK PRACTICE

Those people who practice yoga will know the term 'pranayama' which literally translates as 'expanding the prana' with prana being the vital life force or energy. It is the name given to a number of different types of yogic breathwork exercises.

Even the ancient yogis knew about the connection between breathing and energy generation within our bodies. They also made links between the physical good health that can be generated by correct breathing as well as the mental health benefits and even the spiritual benefits.

There's a whole range of different health benefits associated with correct breathing and breathwork practice so I'll list some of them here.

Strengthening lungs and reducing blood pressure

Regular breathwork exercise should build the capacity of your lungs as well as improve the strength and efficiency of your lung muscles, which in turn will help to boost the health of rest of your body. Your circulatory system should also become more efficient at transferring oxygen to your body's cells and taking away the waste carbon monoxide gas. This can result in lower blood pressure as your circulatory system doesn't need to work so hard to transfer oxygen around the body, with the blood being much more efficiently oxygenated after regular breathwork.

Toning up your body

Regular breathwork exercise makes for a more efficient metabolism and can help to burn excess fat and remove toxins from the body at a faster rate. If you combine breathwork with a good daily exercise routine plus a healthy low-carbohydrate, high-protein diet you could see some amazing results.

Professional athletes normally do some breathwork exercise and this can be useful as both a warm-up exercise as well as for recovering after sport, when it helps to increase the oxygen levels in your blood so that muscle tissue can recover its chemical balance.

Stimulating your digestive system

Breathwork can even help with your digestive system. If the cells in your intestine are better oxygenated they can carry out their task more efficiently, helping to take the energy and digest the nutrients from your food.

Giving you more energy

Because breathwork will make your lungs more effective at capturing oxygen, the individual cells in your body will also get an extra energy boost as they receive more oxygen for respiration. The mitochondria 'battery packs' in your cells will store this extra energy and you should feel a long-term energy boost after a breathwork session.

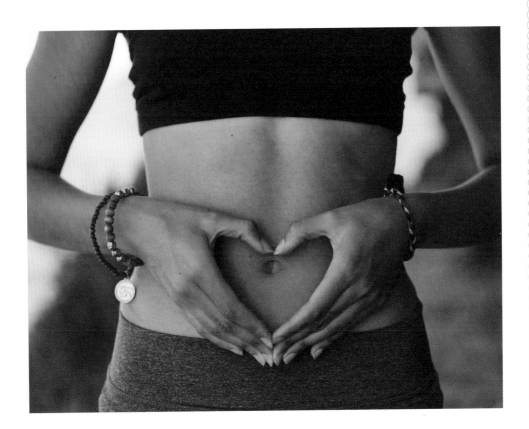

Cleansing your body

As well as speeding up the supply of oxygen to the cells in your body, breathwork also speeds up the removal of toxins such as carbon dioxide from the blood. This can have great health benefits, keeping your individual body cells free of toxins and enabling them to carry out their work more efficiently.

Boosting your mind

The improved flow of oxygen from regular breathwork will also help to keep your brain operating at its optimal level. Oxygen is as essential to the brain as it is to all other parts of the body and we all know about the dangers of oxygen starvation in the brain after something like a stroke. A regular breathwork practice should help you feel more mentally aware and active.

Reducing stress

Staying on the subject of the mind, breathwork can also play an important part in reducing stress. Many meditation techniques start with a concentration on the breath and there are many, simpler breathing exercises that can also help reduce stress in your daily life.

Improving disease resistance

Once you have started to boost your body's absorption of oxygen with breathwork, this can help boost your immune system and lead to many additional health benefits. There are even some specific breathwork exercises that can be used to treat different conditions. For instance, a concentration on breathwork in your nose can help boost your resistance to colds and flu, especially if it is also done alongside regular nasal cleaning, which I will talk about later.

Reducing pain

Breathwork can also boost your body's nervous system, with nerve cells in your spine and throughout your body also benefiting from the increased oxygen supply. Combined with the increased supply of oxygen to the brain this can help to reduce headaches and other body pains.

Helping with menstruation pains

There's even a recognized link between menstruation pain in women and the lining of the nose. In an historic health trial, a gentle application of anesthetic to parts of the nose lining stopped menstruation pain in some women. Without going to this extreme, some breathwork exercises that concentrate on the nose may be helpful for women who suffer from menstrual pain and it's certainly worth trying. Regular nose cleaning may also help here.

Helping with allergies

The nose and the inner nasal cavity are complex structures which carry out a wide range of functions as well as breathing. These include filtering and warming the air as it enters our bodies. There's a natural sneezing reflex to expel a build-up of dust or other irritants in the nose, as well as a swelling of the nasal lining and an extra secretion of mucus to help deal with the problem. If the irritation is severe we may call this a nasal allergy, with perhaps something like pollen or house dust causing the nose to go into overdrive with the production of mucus, as well as the nose lining swelling up and making us sneeze.

Here, breathwork that concentrates on the nose can also be useful, helping you to increase the strength and tolerance of your nasal lining; nasal washing can also help. Breathwork will also build lung strength and give you more of a feeling of control over your entire breathing process which, on its own, can be an important psychological boost for helping to control hay fever.

Helping during panic attacks

When people are having a panic attack and are hyperventilating, one of the recommended aids is to breathe into a paper bag. During hyperventilation, short, sharp, panicked breaths are taken where you exhale too much air and are left with too little carbon dioxide in the blood. This creates an imbalance that also reduces the level of oxygen in the blood. By breathing into a paper bag, the aim is to build up the inhalation of carbon dioxide which helps to restore this balance and should help to reduce the panic. This doesn't work for everyone and isn't recommended for people who suffer from asthma.

If you are someone who suffers from panic attacks, you may find that slow, deep breathing is a better way to stop the attack and regular breathwork practice will help you to prepare for this. Also, regular breathwork exercises can help to reduce panic attacks in the first place, giving you the sense that you are more in control of your breathing.

Helping control and prevent asthma attacks

Breathwork can also have a very positive benefit for those people who suffer from asthma, strengthening your lungs and giving you more control of your breathing so that you feel better able to prevent asthma attacks in the first place. It should also give you more confidence so that you don't panic during an attack and make it worse. This increased confidence may also help to prevent asthma attacks in the first place, since these can sometimes be triggered by the brain on its own, just down to fear and without any external factors such as a pollen or dust mites.

Helping with MS

Breathwork, especially combined with yoga and meditation, can be a help for sufferers of multiple sclerosis. Breathing exercises generally have a positive effect on the nervous system and could help to slow any further degeneration. They can also give sufferers a positive focus and more confidence to help control the disease.

Fighting addiction

Breathwork can even be used as a tool for helping to fight cravings or addiction. Techniques such as rapid abdominal breathing can be used along with yoga and meditation to help give you the strength and willpower and positive mind to break the addiction. It can also give you something new to focus on, as you try and fill the space in your life left by the removal of the addictive substance.

THE RIGHT LEVEL OF BREATHWORK FOR YOU

Although breathwork has many health benefits, there are also some times when it may be best to avoid the more intensive types. I will list here some of the instances when more intensive forms of breathwork may not be suitable. The milder forms of breathwork should be fine for most people but, if in doubt, consult your doctor who will be able to advise what's best for you.

Cardiovascular problems

If you have problems with your heart or other parts of your circulatory system, including high blood pressure, angina or arrhythmia then you should consult your doctor to see if breathwork is suitable for you. Although breathwork has proven health benefits such as stabilizing blood pressure and heart rate, if you have heart problems then really intensive breathwork should be avoided.

History of aneurysms

If you have a family history of aneurysms, there's a very slight risk that the increasing rate of blood circulation and increased blood oxygen levels from intensive breathwork exercises could cause a problem. It's a fairly low risk but consult your doctor for advice if you think this could affect you.

Respiratory problems

If you have a chronic respiratory problem then breathwork may aggravate this so be sure consult your doctor first. For more minor problems, breathwork can be a real benefit as it helps to strengthen the lungs and gives you more control and confidence with your breathing, which can help with conditions like asthma and hay fever.

Pregnancy

Gentle breathwork practice could be beneficial during pregnancy but, as this is a time when your body is dealing with many changes, you don't want to impose too much of a shock on the system with the more intensive forms of breathwork. In addition, really intensive breathwork could also be problematic for those who

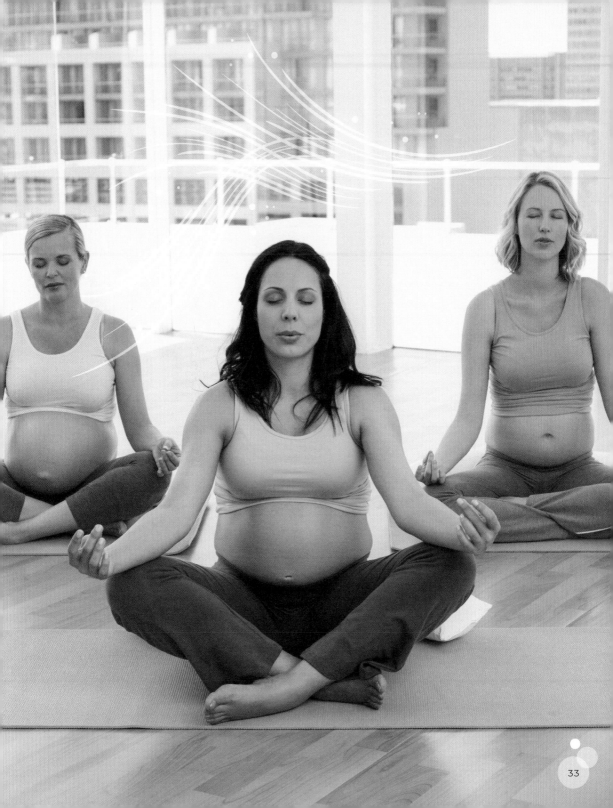

are breast feeding, again because of the shock to the body. Consult your doctor if you plan to do some of the more intensive forms of breathwork.

On medications

You should also check with your doctor if you are taking any strong medications that could conflict with intensive breathwork. Some types of antipsychotic medications, for instance, can be slightly affected if your blood and blood oxygen levels change too much.

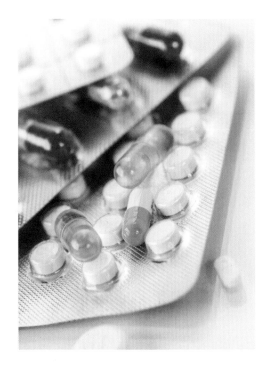

Problems with vision

It's a small risk, but if you suffer from eye conditions such as glaucoma, or have a detached retina, then the rigours of intensive breathwork exercises could be problematic, so consult your doctor or optician first. If intensive breathwork makes you feel too dizzy or affects your vision then you should also avoid this and perhaps have a chat with your doctor.

Risk of seizures

If you have a condition that comes with an increased risk of seizures you should take medical advice before undertaking some of the more advanced and intensive types of breathwork. For some people there's a small risk that boosting the oxygen intake through intensive breathwork exercise could help in triggering a seizure.

Natural side effects

When you are carrying out your breathwork exercises, particularly the more intensive types, there are some natural side effects that can occur, such as dizziness. These shouldn't do you any harm but it's worth knowing about them.

Dizziness

If some breathwork exercises are not practised properly this can lead to a lack of oxygen in the blood, which can result in dizziness and lightheadedness. In most cases, just stopping the exercise and taking slow, deep breaths should reduce this.

Muscle spasms

Intensive breathwork can sometimes cause muscle spasms, in muscles such as the diaphragm or even around your mouth or in your limbs. This is due to the rapid change in oxygen levels and just relaxing for a few minutes and taking slow, deep breaths should resolve this.

Pains in the chest

There's a rare chance that intensive breathwork could cause chest pains, when your respiratory and circulatory systems are put through their paces. In healthy people this should go away if you stop your practice and take slow, deep breaths for a few minutes. If the pains persist then this could be a sign of other health problems, such as a heart condition, so you should consult your doctor.

Blurred vision

If you start to suffer from blurred vision during an intensive breathwork exercise, this again can be due to the rapid change in oxygen levels and should go away if you stop and take slow, deep breaths for a few minutes.

Ringing in the ears

Some people may suffer from ringing in the ears during intensive breathwork, especially if they already suffer from tinnitus or other ear conditions. This again can be due to rapidly changing oxygen levels and increased heart rate. Just stopping to take slow, deep breaths should help to resolve this.

NOSE CLEANSING AS AN AID TO BREATHWORK

Before moving on to describe some of the specific breathwork exercises you can undertake to help boost your health and wellbeing, I think it is important to talk first about the importance of nose cleaning.

Yes, it might sound strange, but nose cleaning is an important part of breathing practice in yoga and has been for many thousands of years. In the language of yoga, this nose-cleansing technique is called 'jala neti', where a small amount of saline water is poured into the nose to cleanse it.

Of course, you don't have to do nose cleansing as part of your breathwork exercises, but it's well worth considering, especially if you often suffer from a blocked nose or nasal infections.

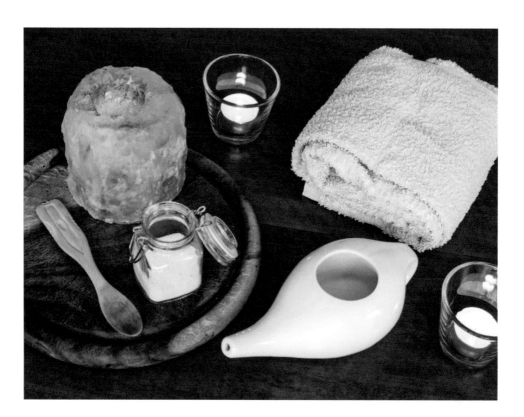

How to clean your nose

The technique of cleaning your nose and nasal cavity is quite simple but for some people it can cause a little apprehension, perhaps with a fear of drowning when it comes to taking water into the nose. If you feel a little worried it may be worth seeking out a qualified yoga teacher who can demonstrate this technique and give you some confidence.

To start, you need to prepare a fairly weak saline solution, perhaps adding a quarter teaspoon or less of salt into a glass or cup of warm water. You can actually buy special nose cleaning cups, called 'neti cups', which have a small spout a bit like a teapot to pour water into each nostril. However, I just use a small glass, something like an alcohol shot glass which has a fairly narrow diameter.

With the glass full of lukewarm, saline water, start by tilting your head back slightly and putting the glass at the end of one nostril. With practice you may be able to let the water flow into one nostril and then back out of the other. However, I personally find it easier to close off one nostril with my finger then pour and gently suck the liquid into the other nostril. If you do this with too much vigor you might force the liquid through your nasal cavity and into the back of your mouth, then down your throat a little, but this is just like having a saltwater mouthwash and won't do any harm.

You actually want the solution to reach into your nasal cavity since here it will flush out dust and pollen, as well as acting to kill bacteria in the nasal cavity.

Once you have poured the solution into one nostril you may need to use some tissue paper to absorb the excess liquid and try to suck this into your mouth and spit it out rather than blowing your nose too much.

Once the liquid flow has settled, swap to your other nostril and repeat the process.

I find that it doesn't take very long for my nose to settle again after cleaning and it's a refreshing feeling to have a moist, fresh nose and nasal cavity afterwards. (Any dog owners will know that a moist dog nose is a sign of good health!)

I tend to do my nasal cleaning first thing in the morning and find that it is a good start to the day, making my nose feel fresh and fluid plus removing any dust and bacteria I may have breathed in during the previous day and overnight.

The benefits of nasal cleansing

Writing this book has encouraged me to increase my own practice of nose cleansing to at least once a day and the benefits have quickly started to show. I now feel that I am breathing more easily and my nose feels more open and free-flowing when I start my breathwork practice.

There are also some great health benefits to be gained from regular nasal cleaning. It helps to remove pollen, dust and other impurities from your nose so can help with allergies such as hay fever and, in some cases, may even help with asthma since these impurities can be a trigger for this.

Perhaps an even bigger benefit is the fact that the salt in the solution used to clean your nose can help kill the bacteria in your nose that can cause colds or other illnesses. It's possible that regular cleaning may also help to flush out viruses and help reduce the chances of catching flu or other respiratory diseases.

As I mentioned earlier, there's also thought to be a link between the lining of the nose and menstruation pains in women. If you suffer from these pains perhaps nasal washing may help a little, keeping the nasal lining in good, clean and healthy condition. There's no hard proof of this but it might be worth trying, as well as undertaking specific breathwork exercises that can help here.

Because the nose and nasal cavity are so closely linked to other parts of the body such as the eyes (via the tear ducts) and even the inner ears (via the eustachian tubes), cleaning your nose and nasal cavity on a regular basis, perhaps along with regular mouth washes, should help prevent infections here as well.

Personally, I feel that my regular nasal-cleaning practice has helped me to breathe more easily, feel fresher and more invigorated at the start of each day, and even reduce headaches. Combined with my breathwork exercises it has created an enhanced feeling of wellbeing and confidence.

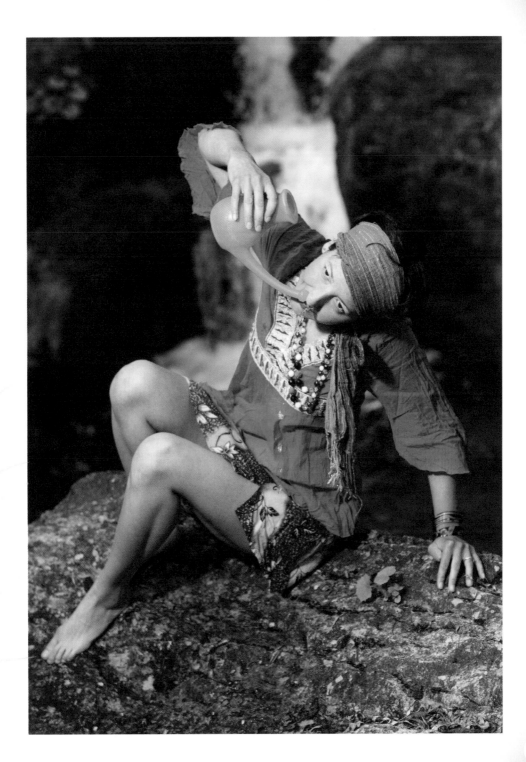

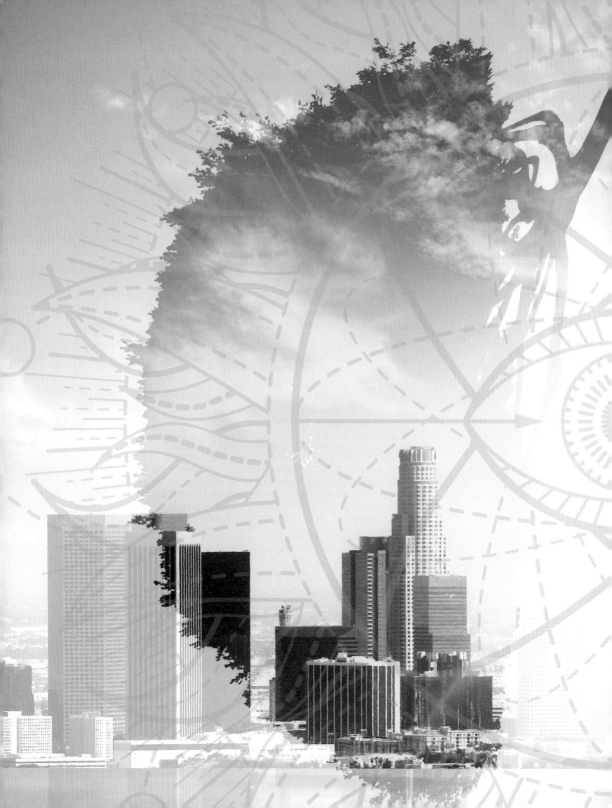

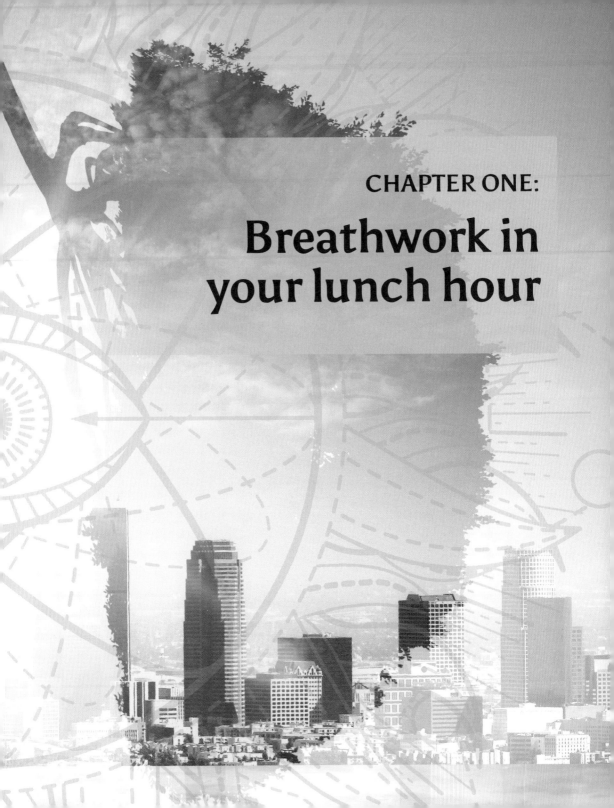

CHAPTER ONE:

Breathwork in your lunch hour

Simple stress-relieving exercises

Breathwork doesn't have to be complex or time-consuming for you to benefit greatly from it, so let's start by looking at some simple exercises which you could carry out at home or even during your lunch hour at work. Any of these would be a good introduction to breathwork, before you move on to more difficult techniques.

EXERCISE 1

Cleansing-breath: to revive and refresh

This is a simple exercise that is designed to cleanse the lungs, stimulate the cells in your body and make you feel revived and refreshed. It can be very helpful for those who have been talking a lot, perhaps spending lots of time on the phone for work.

This forced, vigorous exhalation of air through your narrow mouth opening should give you a refreshed feeling, ready to carry on with the rest of your day in a good mood.

How to practise

In a sitting or standing posture, inhale a complete breath and fill your lungs. As with most breathwork exercises, you should inhale through your nose and not through your mouth.

Hold the air in your lungs for a few seconds, perhaps counting to five in your head.

Then pucker up your lips as if you're about to start whistling and, without expanding your cheeks, exhale about half of the air from your lungs through your puckered mouth in a vigorous way. Stop for a few seconds then vigorously exhale some more of the air. Repeat this process a few times until all the air in your lungs is completely drained.

Once this is done, repeat the process with another breath and continue for five or 10 minutes or more to feel the real benefit.

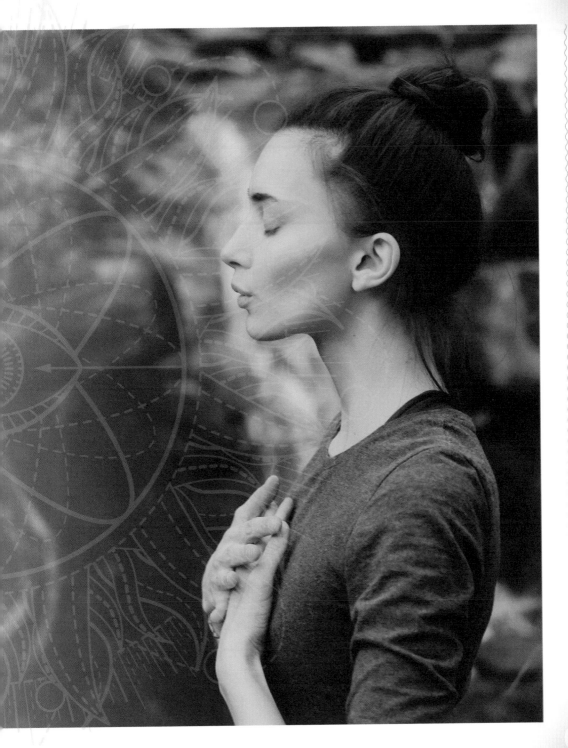

EXERCISE 2

Diaphragmatic breathing: to stimulate your mind and body

Deep, diaphragmatic breathing is one of the most important and basic of all breathwork techniques. Most of us breathe in quite a shallow way, mainly using the intercostal muscles between our ribs to expand the chest and suck in small, shallow breaths. This has the effect of filling the top of the lungs with air but not pushing too much air deep down into the bottom of the lungs.

Due to the force of gravity, the bottom of the lungs is the part heaviest with blood, which in turn carries oxygen from the air to all the cells in our body. With diaphragmatic breathing we breathe in air using the full force of the diaphragm muscle just below our rib cage, which sucks air deep into our lungs so that the maximum amount of oxygen can be passed into the bloodstream, as well as enabling the maximum amount of the waste gas carbon dioxide to be released back in the lungs and exhaled.

This is a technique of breathing that feels a little forced at first but, with regular practice, it becomes more natural and can be very beneficial to our health.

After this type of diaphragmatic breathing, you should feel mentally stimulated and alert, as well as full of energy as your body's cells become fully oxygenated and provide an energy boost.

How to practice

The best way to practise deep, diaphragmatic breathing is to lie flat on your back, perhaps on a yoga mat, though you can also practise it while standing or sitting.

Then, place the palm of one of your hands on the centre of your chest/rib cage. Place the palm of your other hand at the bottom of your rib cage.

Start to slowly inhale deep breaths of air by pulling down on your diaphragm muscle, which contracts and folds flat to suck air into your lungs. With your lower hand, you should feel the base of your chest expanding when you breathe in and your abdomen should rise up.

There should be fairly little movement in the top part of your chest as you breathe this way.

Once you have breathed in, hold the air in your lungs for a second or two, then breathe deeply out using your diaphragm muscle which will be expanding into a dome shape and compressing your lungs as you breathe out.

You can continue this process for perhaps five or 10 minutes to start with but getting longer as you become more used to it.

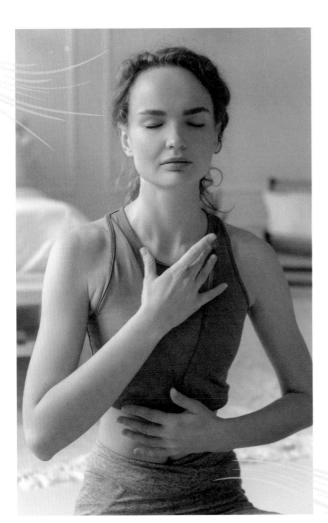

Initially, you may feel a little dizzy as your body takes in much more oxygen than usual, so just stop for a while if you feel like this. With time you will no longer feel dizzy, as your body gets used to this type of deep breathing.

Throughout the exercise you should breathe through your nostrils and not through your mouth. Over time, it is good to slow down your breathing, starting by slowing down your rate of inhalation, taking a bit longer to breathe in, hold your breath for a while, then breathe out slowly as well.

EXERCISE 3
Alternate nostril breathing: to balance and calm nerves

As I mentioned when talking about the nose in an earlier chapter, most of us will naturally be using one nostril more than the other at any particular time when breathing. In effect, one nostril stays in a recovery mode for an hour or so while the other does most of the work, then they naturally swap over.

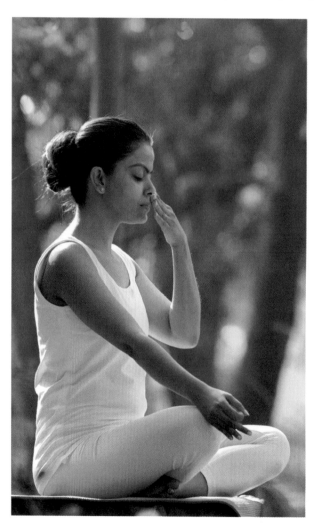

In yoga, each side of the nose is also thought to relate to different parts of the body and mind, in the same way that we sometimes refer to left-brain thinking or right-brain thinking when it comes to people's personalities and abilities.

The practice of alternate nostril breathing, referred to as 'nadi shodhana' by yogis, is one of the fundamental breathing exercises in yoga. By forcing ourselves to use one nostril at a time, then alternating to the other nostril, we are taking time to equalize our breathing and temporarily break the body's natural focus on one particular nostril at any given time.

This creates a balance and stimulates our nervous system, making us feel light and refreshed afterwards. Done in your lunch hour or at other times of day, it should give you a boost and make you feel refreshed to carry on with your day.

How to practise

This type of breathwork is best done in a seated position, either sitting upright in a chair or in a cross-legged yoga posture. When breathing you should take deep, lung-filling breaths and, with experience, you can vary the length of time taken for inhalation, holding your breath and exhalation, mainly by taking longer to hold your breath.

If you are right-handed, hold your hand up to your nose and use the thumb on your right hand to close your right nostril while you breathe in deeply using your left nostril. Hold the breath for a second and then close your left nostril with your third finger, lift your thumb off your right nostril and breathe out fully through your right nostril.

Continue to breathe like this for about 10 breaths and then swap over, so that you breathe in through your right nostril and out through your left nostril.

There are a few variations of this technique and, if you prefer, you can do 10 breaths in and out using the right nostril only, while keeping the left nostril closed, then swap over to do 10 breaths just using the left nostril.

In either case, practice this type of breathing for around five minutes to start with and stop if you start to feel a little dizzy. Over time you can build up to 10 minutes or more.

When you feel confident that you have mastered the technique, you can then add in breath retention. While you are doing the exercise, breathe in slowly and deeply counting up to four in your head, hold the breath in for a count of 16, then exhale during a count of eight.

However much you count to, the desired ratio of time should be 1:4:2 for breathing in, holding your breath, and then exhaling.

EXERCISE 4

Crocodile-pose breathing: to help you really tune into and feel your breathing

When we are beginners to breathwork exercise, it can take a while to understand exactly how much work the body does when breathing. This exercise involves lying on your front, so your belly and chest press against the floor when breathing and you really feel the expansion of your chest.

How to practise

Lie down on the floor on your front, using a yoga mat or other cushioned mattress to support you. Fold your arms and place them under your head, so that your forehead rests on them. With your arms crossed under your head, the top of your chest should be slightly lifted off the floor. Also, spread your legs out a comfortable distance apart and with your toes facing outwards.

Start to slowly inhale deep breaths of air by pulling down on your diaphragm muscle. You should feel your chest expanding and pushing against the floor when you breathe in.

Once you have breathed in, hold the air in your lungs for a count of two or three in your head, feeling how your abdomen is pressed against the floor. Then breathe deeply out using your diaphragm muscle to force all the air out of your lungs. You should feel your abdominal muscles relaxing and less pressure on your abdomen as it shrinks away from the floor.

You can continue this process for five minutes or so, even starting to regulate your inhalations and exhalations if you want to increase the intensity. To do this, try counting to three during inhalation, holding your breath for a count of two, then exhaling during a count of four.

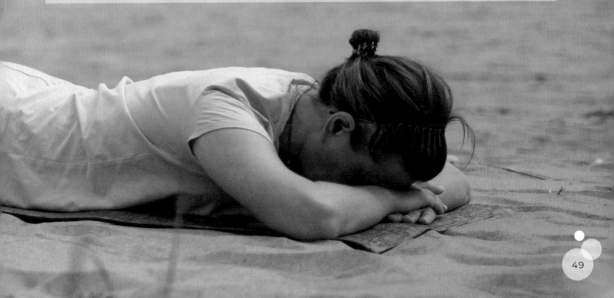

EXERCISE 5
Walking breath: a simple breathwork exercise to practise if you go outside in your lunch break

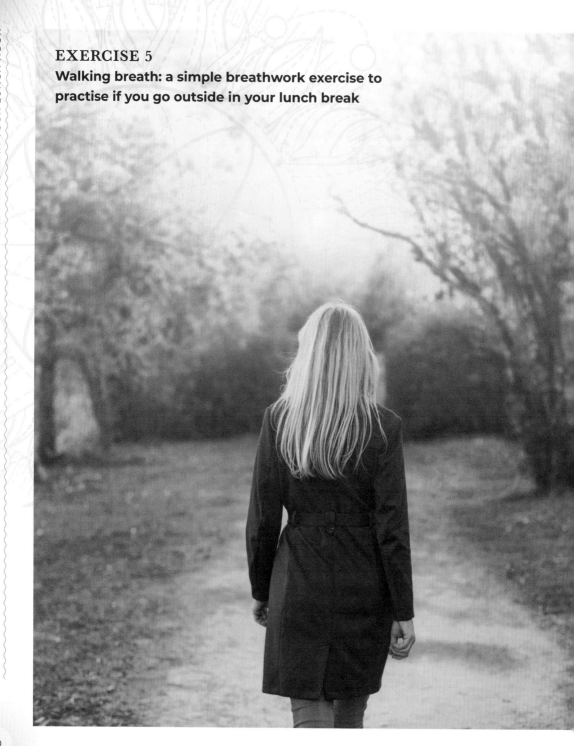

If you work in an office, factory or any other indoor environment, it can be good to get out for a short walk in your lunch hour, to exercise your body and refresh your mind, as well as perhaps stopping to grab a sandwich somewhere.

This breathwork exercise allows you to use this time in an even more constructive way, helping to calm your mind and remove some of the stresses of the day, as well as gradually strengthening your lungs.

How to practise

Walk along at your normal pace but start to focus on your breath. How many steps do you complete during each inhalation and exhalation? You'll probably find it's only a couple of steps for each inhalation and exhalation.

Now try to extend the number of steps you take during each inhalation and exhalation, by slowing down your breathing rather than walking faster. Set yourself the target of four steps during each inhalation and four steps during each exhalation. You might find it a bit strange at first to concentrate on your walking and breathing like this, a bit like a child walking along and trying to avoid the cracks in the pavement.

Keep this breathwork exercise up for the duration of the walk, or as long as you are able.

As you get used to this, after a few days try to increase the number of steps you take during each inhalation and exhalation, aiming for six steps. Then, once you have become used to this, increase it to eight steps during each inhalation and each exhalation.

Once you get to eight steps, this will probably be getting close to the limit of what is comfortable and, of course, if you feel dizzy at any point just stop for a minute or so to recover, breathing deeply and slowly.

You should feel very refreshed afterwards and the focus on breathing should help to remove some of the stress and tensions that may have built up during your morning at work.

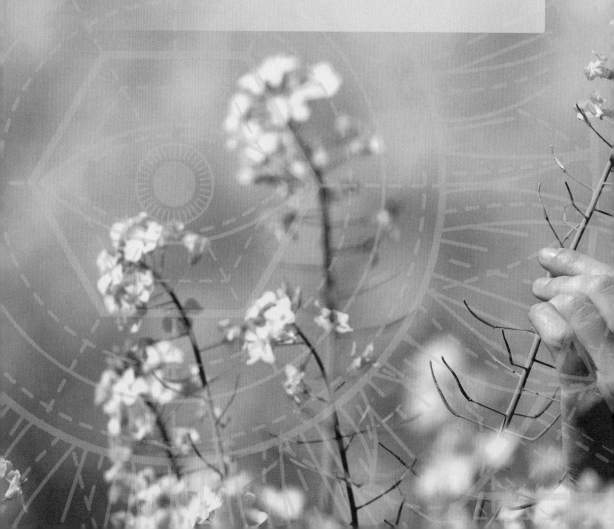

CHAPTER TWO

Breathwork for leisure

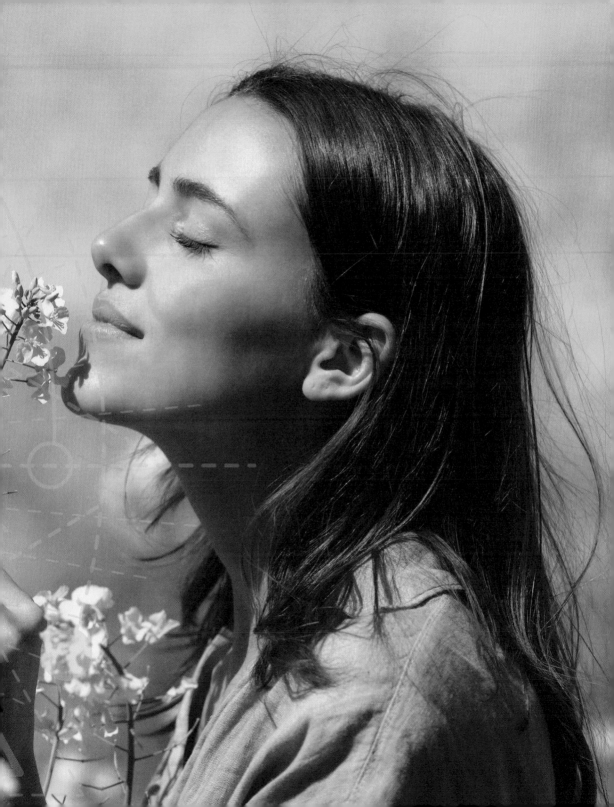

With more time to devote to your practice

Perhaps the best time to start your breathwork practice is when you are feeling relaxed and have some time on your hands. This could be during a holiday from work, or just over a weekend, when you are free from your regular routines and have time to dedicate to breathwork.

Any of the previous exercises would be suitable of course, but here I will give you some slightly more complex breathing exercises that can involve different postures or last for longer periods of time.

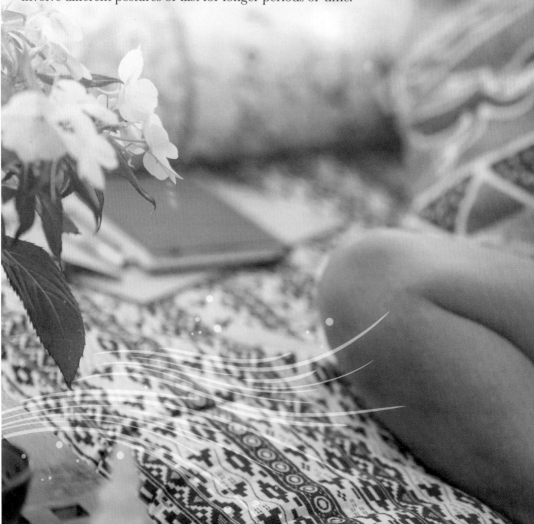

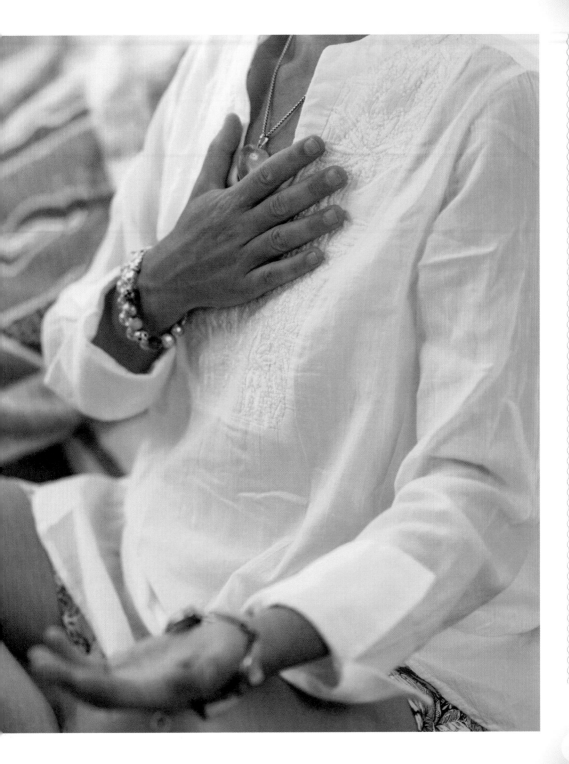

EXERCISE 6
Weighted chest breathing: to achieve a relaxed, restful state

For this breathwork exercise you will need something like a yoga mat that you can lie down on, as well as a soft weight of some sort, such as a sandbag or weighted cushion, up to about three or four pounds in weight.

The idea of this technique is to practice deep, rhythmic, diaphragmatic breathing by feeling your chest rising up with each inhalation then lowering with each exhalation.

It will help to strengthen your abdominal muscles and your diaphragm as well as fully oxygenating all parts of your body, giving you a feeling of health and wellbeing and putting you into a relaxed state.

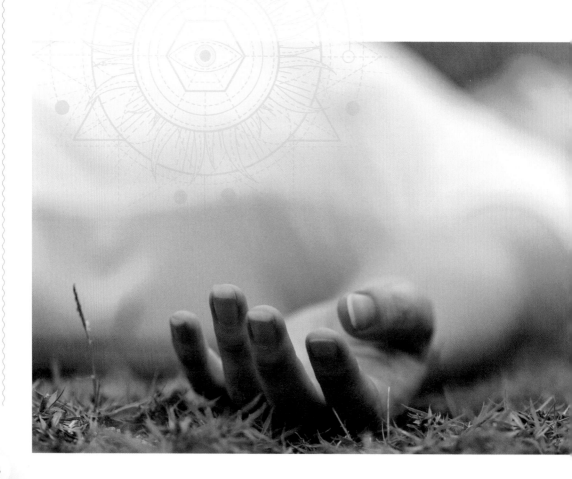

How to practise

Using either a yoga mat or some other soft floor surface, lie on your back with your legs and arms spread comfortably apart. For extra comfort you may also want to use a shallow neck pillow or even a thin pillow under the small of your back if you have back problems.

Close your lips gently and take a few moments to relax your body from head to toe, then place the small sandbag or similar weight onto your abdomen, at the bottom of your ribcage.

Close your eyes and start breathing steadily and deeply. You should feel the sandbag rise as you inhale and fall back as you exhale. The sandbag means that you will have to make more effort when inhaling, but exhaling should be effortless.

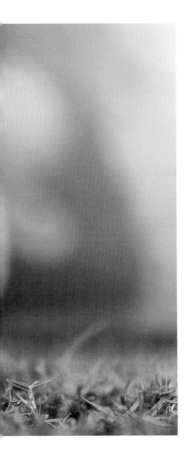

You may want to hold your breath for a second or two but generally the aim is to make breathing as rhythmic as possible, with the same time given to inhalation and exhalation.

To start with, carry out this breathing practice for five minutes or so at a time and then remove the sandbag and relax for a few more minutes before turning onto your side and slowly getting up off the floor.

If you have plenty of free time, such as during a holiday, leave your yoga mat out on the floor and do this exercise several times each day. Once you are used to it, try to elongate the time taken for each exhalation and inhalation.

If you continue breathwork exercise over several weeks, assimilating it into your daily routine, you should feel a sense of deep relaxation each time, calming your nerves. It should also help to boost your general health, since many illnesses, both physical and mental, are made worse by too much stress in our lives.

EXERCISE 7

Sounds breathing: to bring back those good vibrations

Now we are going to start making some noise, so this is definitely a breathwork exercise that will not go down well in your office lunch hour, but could be perfect if you're enjoying a holiday somewhere or are at home.

Making sounds when you breathe out causes vibrations that stimulate your whole body and bring your voice box into action. If you've sung along at a pop concert, or belted out hymns during a religious service, you'll know just how invigorating and stimulating this can be and how you often feel much happier afterwards.

Breathwork exercises that use sound can have a similar effect. As well as oxygenating your blood, you're also invigorating your whole body as well as stimulating your mind. It can be a really refreshing experience and, even if you start coughing a little afterwards, this is just your body removing phlegm which it wants to do anyway.

How to practise

Put yourself in a comfortable seated position, either on a chair or in a cross-legged or kneeling posture on the floor. However you sit, make sure your back is kept straight and you're not putting any part of your body in an awkward or uncomfortable position.

Take a deep breath in through your nose and then exhale through your mouth making a continual and loud 'ahhh' sound. Feel the vibrations spread throughout your body, from your head to your toes, and don't hold back if you feel like being really loud.

Repeat this process three times and then change so that you make a continual 'oooo' sound instead, as you breathe out. Again, do this three times and feel the vibrations throughout your body.

Finally, change to a continual 'mmmm' sound as you breathe out, closing your lips to make this sound. Also do this three times.

Finally, combine all three sounds in one word as you breathe out, making the sound 'ahhhooommm' and closing your lips with the final 'mmm'. Also do this three times.

You can then repeat the whole process as many times as you want, but five to 10 minutes would be a good time to practise this breathwork exercise.

These three sounds when added together form the most fundamental of yoga and meditation chants in the form of the word 'om' which is pronounced more like 'ahhhooommm' when used as a mantra or chant.

In Yoga, 'om' is seen as the origin seed or 'bija', the most fundamental sound in the universe, from which all other sounds stem.

By making this sound you are connecting with the vibrations of the universe, forming an invigorating breathwork exercise that can also make you more mentally aware and help to develop your spiritual side.

EXERCISE 8

Three-section breathing: to help you control your body and mind

One of the main principles behind breathwork exercises when used in yoga or for meditation is to put you in control of your own breathing and by extension more in control of your whole body. The bodily function of breathing is automatic, happening without us even thinking about it. However, breathwork exercise gives us the chance to manipulate our breathing, controlling both it and the effects that it has on the rest of our body, including our organs and our nervous system.

This three-section breathing exercise is all about control, making you control and feel all the parts of your body involved with breathing. Your diaphragm muscle, intercostal chest muscles (which run between your ribs) and your collarbone muscles are the three main muscles used in breathing. This breathing technique concentrates on each muscle in turn, so you can feel how each plays its part in the breathing process and you will gain more control of your breathing.

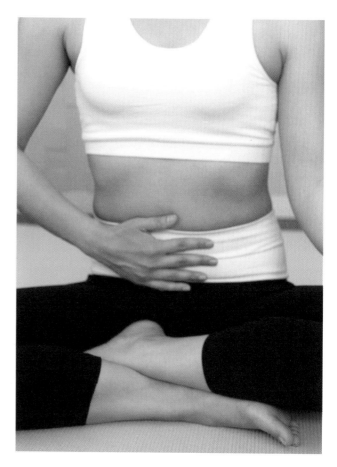

This will lead to a greater understanding of your body, helping you with all the other breathwork exercises you may undertake.

On a wider level, this exercise should help you to feel in control of your life, putting you back in touch with your body and grounding your mind, helping to reduce stress in your life. You should feel invigorated and have more drive to change the things in your life that you are not happy with.

How to practise

Put yourself in a comfortable seating position, either on a chair or in a cross-legged yoga pose, or perhaps kneeling if you prefer this.

Place one of your hands on your abdomen and concentrate on keeping your shoulders and upper chest as stationary as possible, then inhale deeply through your nose, using your diaphragm muscle. Use your hand to feel your abdomen bulge. Then exhale through your nose by drawing in your abdomen slowly and steadily, feeling the contraction with your hand.

Next it is time to feel your intercostal chest muscles at work. Move your hands so that your palms are on each side of your rib cage and keep your shoulders and abdomen as still as possible. Then breathe in by expanding your rib cage. Feel your ribs expand apart from each other as you inhale. Then exhale by contracting your rib cage. In the final stages of exhalation you can also use the palms of your hands to push on the sides of your rib cage and help to expel the last of the air. This will also help you to feel the intercostal muscles in action.

The final stage of this exercise is to breathe using our collarbone and shoulders. This is part of the breathing process that is normally only used when we are really out of breath, such as at the end of a marathon run when you'll often see runners with their shoulders going up and down as they take in as much breath as possible.

If you want to feel your shoulders rising during this type of inhalation you could touch your shoulders with your hands for the first few breaths and see how they move. It will feel quite strange at first, just raising your shoulders and collarbone to inhale air, plus you won't be taking in as much air as before. Once you have fully raised your shoulders and taken in air, lower your collarbone and shoulders to exhale the air. You'll probably get the sensation of air leaving when you breathe out this way, but not much sensation of the more limited amount of air entering your lungs.

Finally, it's time to combine all three types of breathing on a single breath. Start by inhaling using your abdomen, then continue by switching to your chest muscles, then finally bring in your shoulder and collarbone muscles. Then exhale by reversing the order, starting by lowering your collarbone and shoulder muscles.

It's a breathing exercise that needs a lot of concentration, especially when you combine the three different types of breathing at the end, but it's worth continuing until you have mastered it.

You can also spread the process out, giving you more time to perfect each step. So, perhaps do 10 breaths concentrating on your abdomen, then 10 concentrating on your chest, then 10 using your shoulder and collarbone muscles. Finally bring them all together with 10 of the combined breaths.

To start with, five minutes should be enough for this exercise but you can later make it longer or combine it with other breathwork exercises.

EXERCISE 9
Folded tongue breathing: to stimulate the senses and help with digestive problems

This breathwork exercise is used by yogis to focus on the mouth and tongue and is thought to help with illnesses such as a cold or sore throat, plus is also seen as good for digestion and the digestive system in general.

It is a fairly simple exercise so would be great as part of a regular routine alongside other breathwork practice.

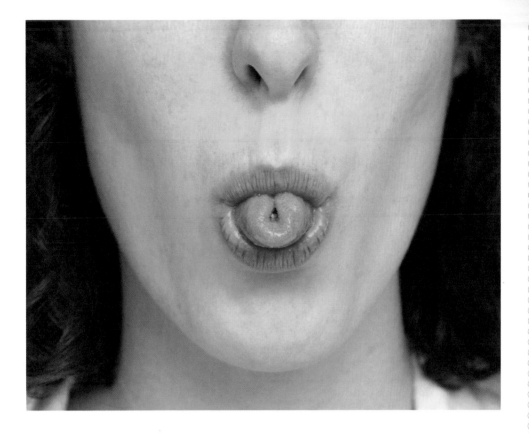

How to practise

Sit in a comfortable position, either in a chair or on the floor. Then twist your tongue so that it forms a tube-like channel in your mouth.

Breathe in through your mouth slowly and feel the air pass down and around the tube of your tongue and into your lungs. Take a full, deep breath and then close your mouth before breathing out through your nose.

Repeat the process for five minutes or so and vary things by holding your breath in for a few seconds before you exhale, plus take time to experience the inflow of air as it surrounds your tongue.

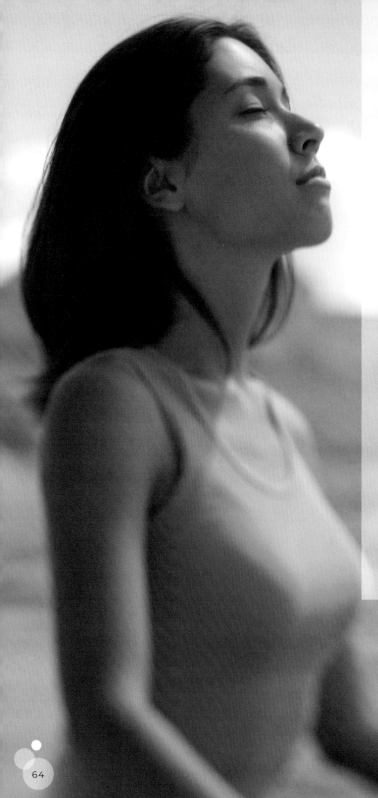

EXERCISE 10
Holding the breath, or Kumbaka, breathing: for calmness and relaxation

This breathwork exercise involves changing the ratio between the time taken to breath in and breathe out, while holding in your breath for a period of time. By holding in your breath you become still for a few seconds, helping to calm your mind and giving you plenty to focus on rather than letting your mind wander and think about all the stress in your life. It can be practiced at any time of day, but doing it just before you go to bed should help you to relax and get ready for sleep.

How to practise

Get yourself into a comfortable seated position, either cross-legged in a yoga posture with your hands on your knees and palms facing up, or on your knees, or even in a chair. Make sure your back is straight, head is up and your shoulders are relaxed and down. Your arms and hands should also be relaxed.

Breathe in slowly through your nose, counting until five in your head.

Then, hold your breath in for another count of five, keeping your shoulders relaxed and your spine feeling straight and long, noticing how full your lungs feel.

Then, breathe out slowly through your nose for another count of five, again keeping your shoulders relaxed and back straight.

Do this five times and then relax for a few seconds. You should have a feeling of lightness as well as feeling stable and grounded.

This is like a warm-up and the next step is to increase the duration of the held breath. So, breathe in for a count of five, then hold your breath in for a count of 10, before exhaling very slowly and deliberately for a count of 10.

Do this between five and 10 times then relax for a few seconds before doing some more. Three or four sets should be enough to help you relax.

Once you have mastered this technique, you should increase the period of holding in your breath for a count of 15 seconds. You can vary the timings if you want, but try to maintain the ratio of 1:3:2 for the time taken to breathe in, hold your breath and exhale. So, for instance, that could be a count of four when inhaling, a count of 12 when holding the breath, then a count of eight during exhalation.

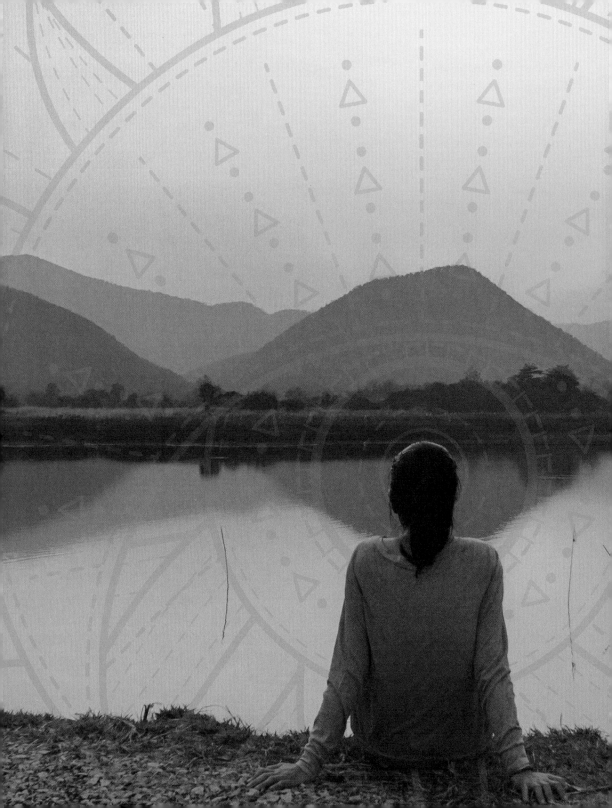

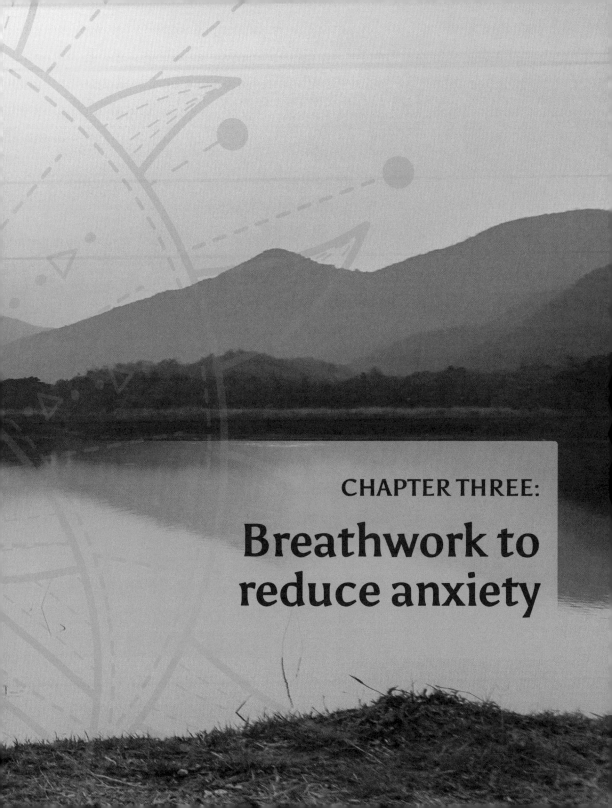

CHAPTER THREE:

Breathwork to reduce anxiety

Helping you to recover from the stresses and strains of the day

Most of the breathwork exercises in this book will be useful to help reduce anxiety and stress but here are a few that may be particularly good. Breathwork also plays a big part in many meditation practices, with a concentration on breathing often used as a way to guide people into a meditative state. If you don't already do it, I would say it's well worth thinking about meditation practice in the future, which can also help to reduce your stress levels.

EXERCISE 11

Throat vibration breathing: a noisy exercise to help chase off stress and anxiety

This exercise makes use of your tongue and is also good for releasing the tension around your head and neck, helping to remove feelings of stress. It can even help if you are suffering from a cold or sore throat.

How to practise

Sit in the classic, cross-legged yoga pose, with your hands resting on your knees and palms facing upwards. Inhale normally through your nose, hold your breath for a second, then open your mouth and stick your tongue out as far as it will go, trying to touch your chin. Tuck your chin in as far as you can so that it is pressing slightly against your throat. Keep your shoulders relaxed and also fully open the palms of your hands and stretch out the soles of your feet. Also make your eyes look upwards, as if focusing

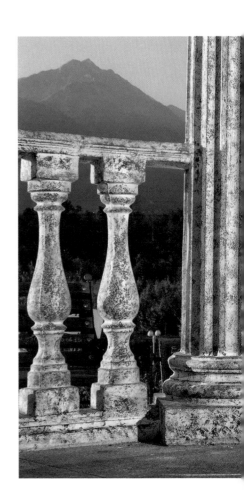

on a point between your eyebrows. Then exhale strongly, trying to extend your tongue all the time.

You should feel a vibration in your throat as you exhale, making a roaring sound, and you can make this as loud as possible.

You can repeat this breath four or five times but it's a strong exercise so you won't be able to do it for too long. Your throat might start hurting after a while if you overdo this exercise.

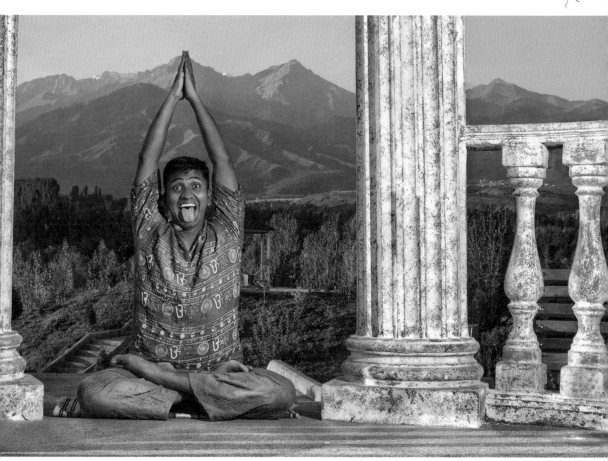

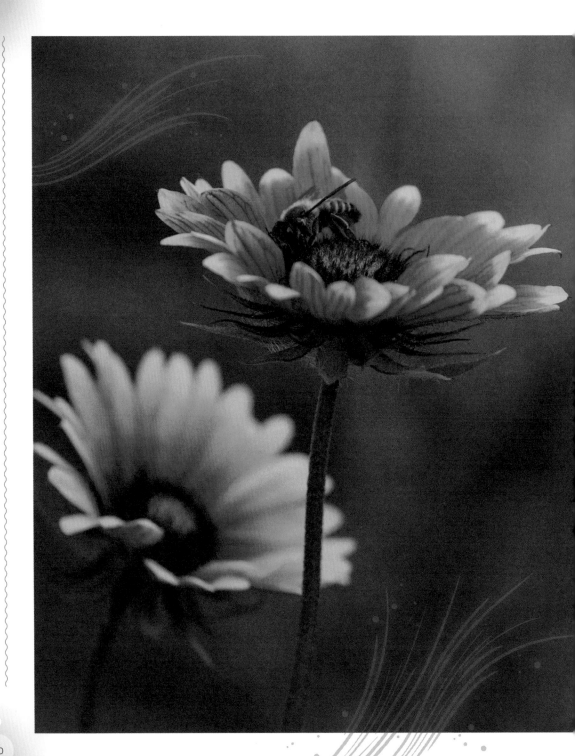

EXERCISE 12
Bee vibration breathing: a noisy way to reduce stress

This simple exercise might make a lot of noise, as you hum like a buzzing bee, but it's a very calming type of breathwork and you should feel very relaxed and refreshed afterwards. It's good for relaxing your shoulders and neck and can help you to sit correctly, adopting a pain-free posture.

How to practise

Sit in a comfortable, cross-legged yoga pose, with your palms resting on your knees and facing upwards; you can sit on a chair if you prefer. Make sure you are sitting properly upright, with an elongated, flat spine and straight neck.

Start by inhaling and exhaling slowly through your nose for a few breaths, keeping your shoulders relaxed. Then, take a deeper breath in, gently close your lips, and exhale through your mouth so that your lips gently vibrate as the air leaves.

One of the main parts of this exercise is to experience and really feel the bee-like vibrations as you exhale. Feel the vibration on the back of your neck and running down your straight spine. You may also feel the vibration in your ribcage. Feel the buzzing slow down as you exhale the last of the air and get ready for a fresh inhalation.

Enjoy the feeling of sitting bolt upright and sensing the buzzing throughout your body.

It's best to do this exercise in small sets, perhaps with 10 breaths in and out, then stop for a while before doing another 10 breaths. Something like three sets should be enough, but do more if you feel you're getting a real buzz from this exercise.

It's a loud, active and buzzing breathwork exercise, but in the stillness afterwards you should feel fresh, awake and very relaxed, ready for the rest of your day.

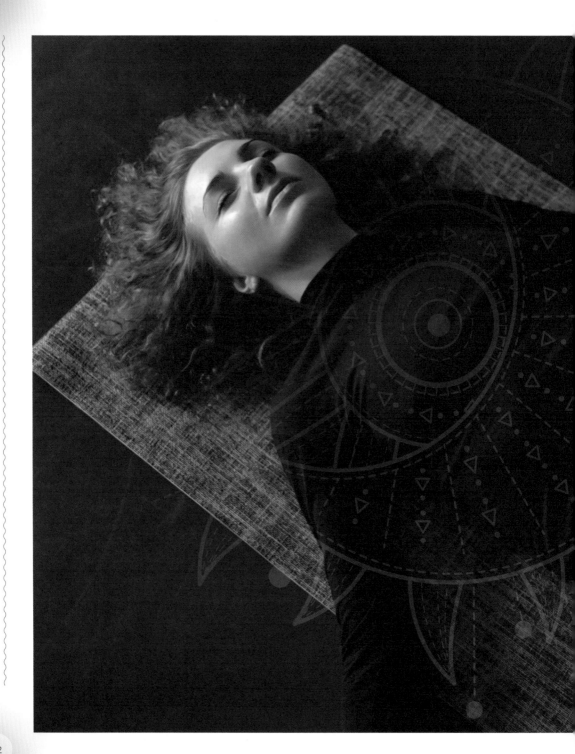

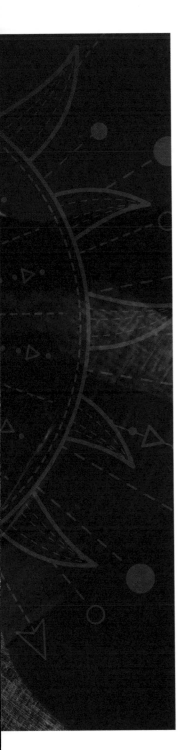

EXERCISE 13
Square breathing: to reduce stress and help stop hyperventilation during a panic attack

This breathwork practice is often called 'square breathing' as it involves four counts of four during the exercise. Yogis often refer to this as Sama Vritti breathing. It can help reduce stress and even help to prevent hyperventilation during a panic attack. It can also help improve your sleep, so could be something to practise in the evening before you go to bed.

How to practise

Find a comfortable position, either sitting, standing or lying down.

Take a deep and slow breath in through your nose, filling your lungs, and continue inhaling for a silent count of four.

Then hold the breath in your lungs for another count of four, before slowly exhaling during another count of four. Then, hold your lungs empty for a count of four, before repeating the whole process.

I would suggest sets of 10 breaths like this, before resting for a minute and then starting another set of 10, perhaps with three sets in total.

If you suffer from panic attacks, learning a slow-paced, controlled breathing exercise like this could be great for when an attack happens, though you will need some strength of mind to start practising it in the middle of an attack. However, just knowing that you have the ability to control an attack might be a psychological boost to help prevent them in the first place.

EXERCISE 14
Equal breath breathing: to calm and focus your mind

This is a very simple breathwork technique which might be a good starting point if you are new to breathwork or have limited free time in your busy day to try and de-stress and focus your mind. It can also help you to relax when getting ready for bed at night.

How to practise

This exercise can be done in a seated or standing position, but in either case make sure your back is straight and your shoulders are relaxed and down before you start.

Spend a couple of minutes just focusing on your normal, nasal breathing, without changing it. Focus on the sensation of your lungs expanding and contracting and of the air entering your nose and flowing into your lungs.

Then, breathe in deeply through your nose for a count of four in your head. Once your lungs are full, exhale through your nose for another count of four, emptying your lungs.

Continue taking these equal breaths for five minutes or more, all the while focusing on how the air feels as it enters and leaves your body.

EXERCISE 15
Mantra breathwork: adding a mantra to your breathwork, for added focus on relaxation

A mantra is a repeated word or set of words which are often used in meditation practice, where they play an important part in focusing the mind and taking your thoughts away from everyday life.

Without going into a full meditative state, you can still use mantras as part of a breathwork practice, where they will also help to focus the mind and make you feel calmer and more relaxed afterwards, perhaps ready for sleep if it's bedtime.

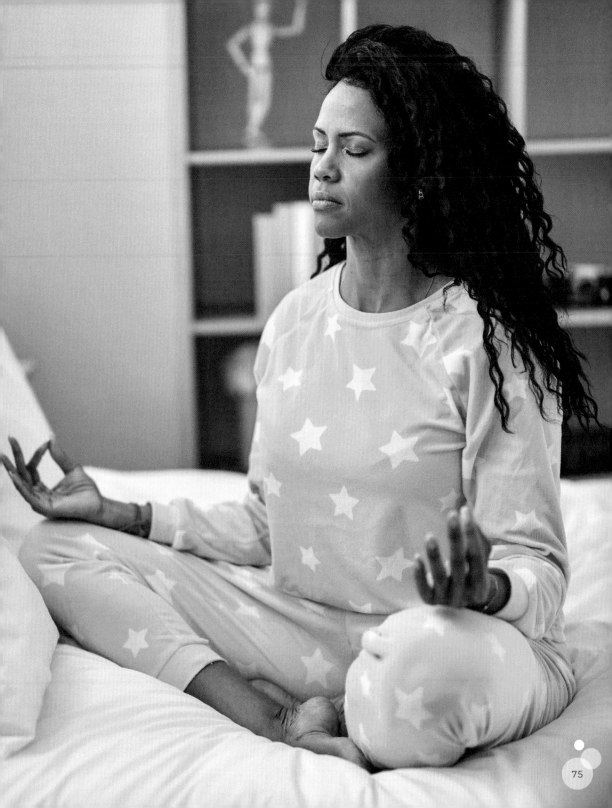

How to practise

Either lie down on your back or find a comfortable seated position.
If you are seated make sure your back is straight and your shoulders
are lowered and relaxed. If in a lying position, make sure you are
comfortable with your lower back and legs supported on small
cushions if you like.

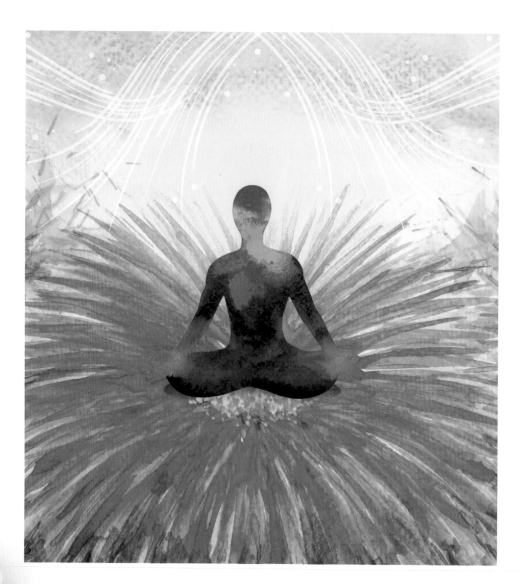

Begin by breathing in deeply through your nose, using your chest muscles and diaphragm muscle to pull air down into the depths of your lungs. Breathe in slowly for a period of five seconds and, while you do so, repeat a mantra in your head which could be something simple like, 'take energy'.

Then, hold your breath for a second before exhaling all the air from your lungs through your nose slowly and steadily for another five seconds. While doing this repeat another mantra in your head, which could be something like 'remove stress'.

Do this 10 times then go back to normal breathing for a minute or so, before repeating.

You can also use this mantra technique to help you deal with specific forms of stress in your life, just by changing the mantra to something that has a specific meaning to you. For instance, if you want to regain your self-confidence after a relationship break-up, you could inhale using the mantra 'love life' then exhale with the mantra 'free from him/her'. You could even use mantras in breathwork to mentally help with illnesses, perhaps with something like 'breathing strength' when you inhale and 'rejecting illness' when you exhale, perhaps naming the particular illness in the mantra.

It might sound odd, but this use of simple mantras can really help to create a positive attitude and empower you to deal with problems in your life. Increasingly, even doctors and others in the medical profession are realizing the power of the mind when it comes to fighting illness, with positive thinking being as good as medicine in some cases.

Just think of all those medical trials where the placebo works almost as well as the real drug, just because people have the positive perception that they are getting better.

EXERCISE 16

Breathing with images: to focus your mind away from daily stress and anxiety

If you have time to lie down for a few minutes, either on a bed or a yoga mat, this exercise can really help you to de-stress and focus your mind away from things that may be bothering you. It can also be good at nighttime, when you are trying to relax and get off to sleep.

How to practise

Lie down on your back, on a bed or yoga mat, making sure you feel comfortable, with your neck, lower back and legs supported on small cushions if this helps.

Close your eyes and start to focus on your breath, focusing on how relaxed and comfortable you feel when you exhale.

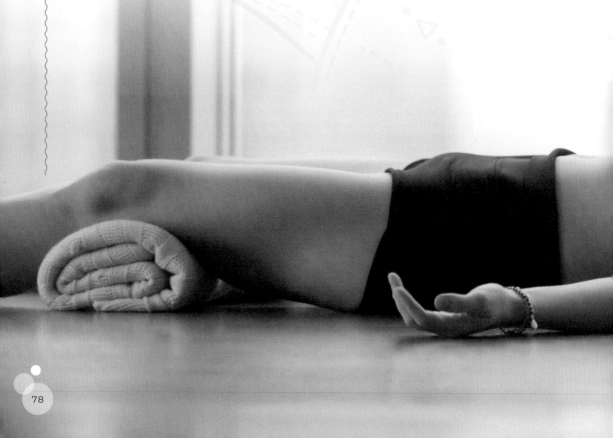

Then start to take slightly deeper breaths, through your nose, holding in your breath for a couple of seconds before exhaling completely. Again, focus on your body as you exhale through your nose, how your weight is pushing down into the mattress and how the mattress or floor is supporting your body.

Now, with each slow exhalation of air, focus less on your body and think about a pleasant image to represent the air as it flows out. Perhaps think of this air as your favourite colour. So, for instance, imagine yourself exhaling bright blue air. You could also think of perfume smells, or flower petals, imagining that you are exhaling these out into the world. Let your imagination run away with you, to find an image that you really like.

Carry on breathing gently like this for as long as you like; you might even fall asleep in the process!

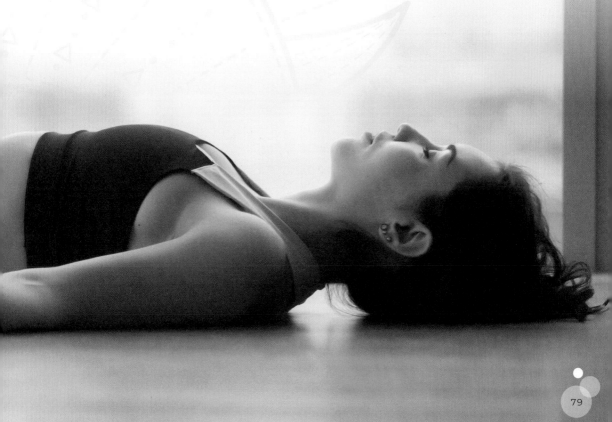

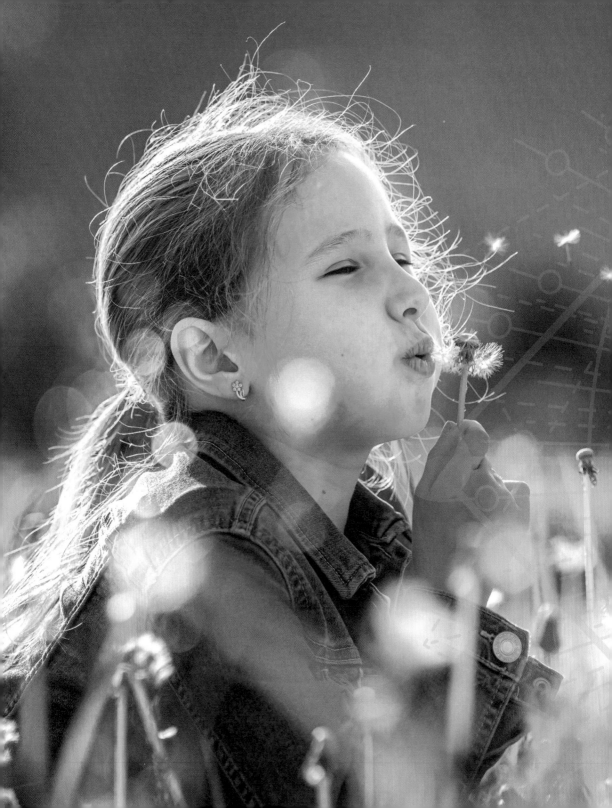

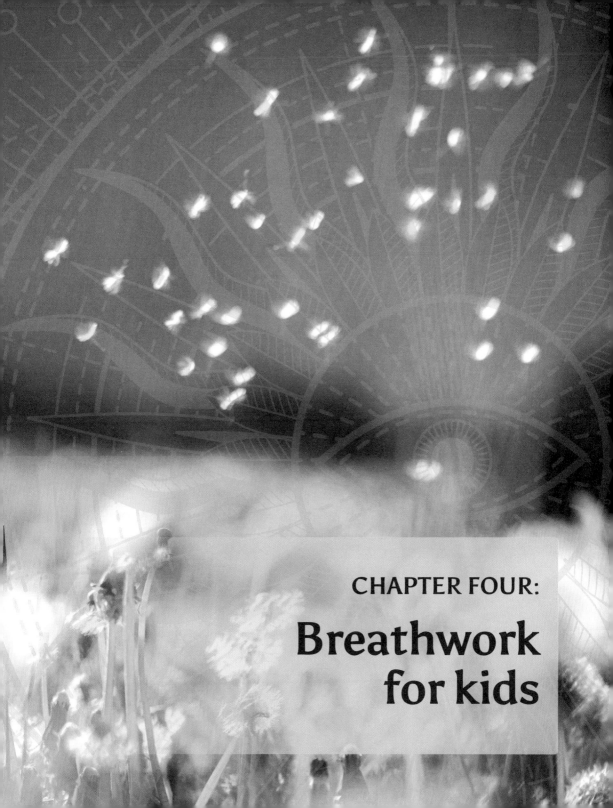

CHAPTER FOUR:

Breathwork for kids

Make it fun and help them to strengthen their lungs

If you've got young children and they see you huffing and puffing in the corner of the room doing your breathwork exercises, they are bound to want to join in. So, why not do some simple and fun breathwork exercises with them?

We've got a few easy exercises here which kids should enjoy and which could also benefit them, especially if they suffer from respiratory problems such as hay fever or even a milder type of asthma. Even though these are fairly mild breathing exercises it's probably best to consult your doctor first if your child has more serious respiratory problems.

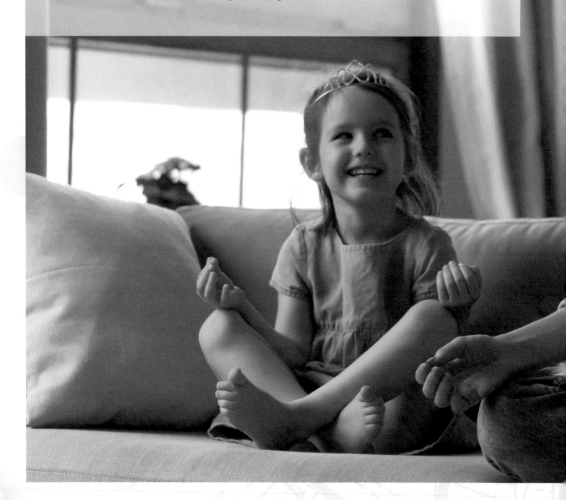

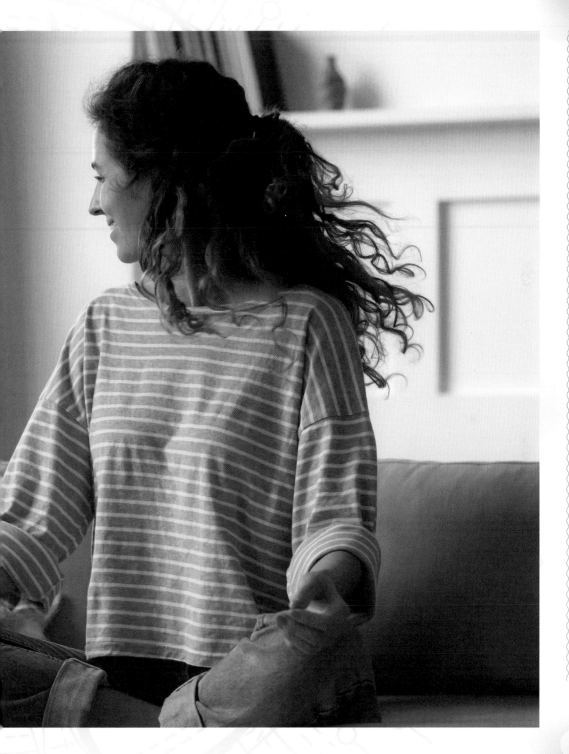

EXERCISE 17
Discovering your breath: simple exercises to help kids think about their breathing

Just making children aware of their breath and how it works can give them a focus and calm them down for a few minutes. You might also want to explain the basic biology of breathing to kids before you start, telling them how air and oxygen is as important for our bodies as food and water.

How to practise

If it's a cold day, a simple exercise to start with is to sit your child in front of a window or mirror and get them to take a deep breath and then breathe out though their mouth onto the window. Show them how the moisture in their breath is making a mist on the window. They can even make shapes with their fingers in this mist and this can become a game in itself.

Then tell them to breathe in, purse their lips, and breathe out quickly onto the window as if trying to cool down hot food. They should notice how much less mist there is when cold breath like this is quickly exhaled.

After this you can continue with another exercise to make children aware of their breathing. Get them to lie on the floor on their backs and place their hands on their bellies. Tell them to breathe in deeply and feel their bellies expanding as they inhale deep into their lungs. Ask them if their belly feels like a balloon that is being blown up and tell them to continue breathing in and out, using nothing but air to make their tummies rise up and down.

By doing this exercise you are encouraging children in deep, diaphragmatic breathing to strengthen their lungs, at the same time educating them on how breathing works.

A similar exercise can be done if you ask a child to sit with their back touching a wall and then ask them to breathe deeply, feeling how their back grows against the wall when inhaling and falls back when exhaling. Tell the child to imagine their back is covered in paint and to think about what sort of mark this would make on the wall when they breathe in, expanding their chest and back. You can even sit two kids back-to-back and ask them to feel each other's breathing against their backs.

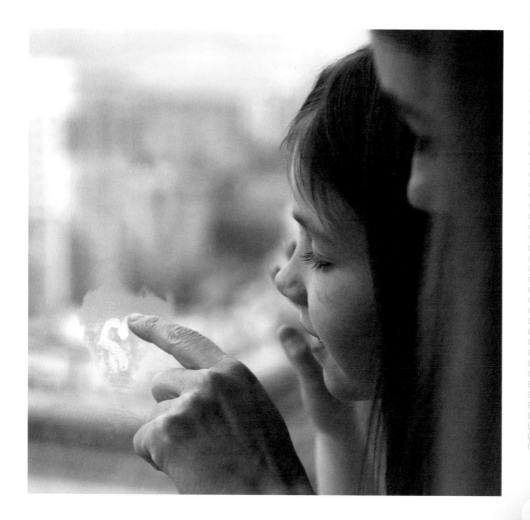

EXERCISE 18
Animal breathing: make fun animal sounds to explore your breathing

Most children have a love of animals and some of the more serious breathwork practices actually encourage animal-like sounds when breathing out, such as making the buzzing noise of a bee. This creates vibrations in your body which complement the breathwork.

So, this simple breathing exercise actually encourages children to make animal noises. You should also have fun practising it with them.

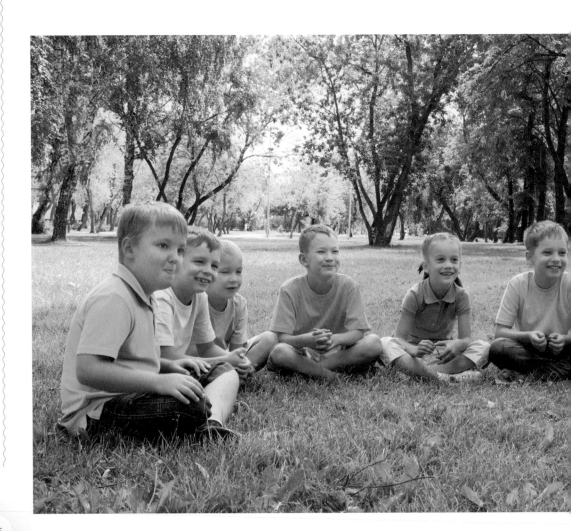

How to practise

You can do this exercise either seated cross-legged on the floor or standing up, even wandering around the room if you've got a load of active toddlers to keep happy.

Tell the child or children to pretend they are part of a swarm of bees, flying between flowers in the garden. Tell them to breathe in through their noses and then breathe out using their mouth, tongue and lips to make the buzzing sound of the bee. They can even run round the room with their arms out, pretending to fly like a bee.

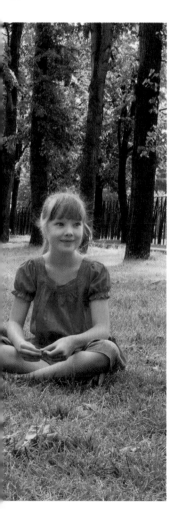

If they want to try another animal, suggest something big and dangerous like a lion or tiger. Tell them to get on all fours and walk round the room making a roaring sound, moving their heads around and looking menacing. Ask them afterwards if they could feel this roar giving them a rough sensation in their throats. Explain that their own voices also come from down in their throats as the air coming out is manipulated by their voice box.

Then, what about something to help them practise whistling? Get them to sit down and pretend to be a wise owl. Tell them to put one hand on their stomach so they can feel air going in and out then ask them to inhale and close their lips into a small circle before breathing out and making a 'twit twoo' whistling owl sound, or just a single-note bird sound if they prefer. If you've got a few kids in a group, tell them to get louder and louder each time and watch them compete with each other and have fun.

At the end, ask them if there are any other animal sounds they want to make, to encourage their creativity.

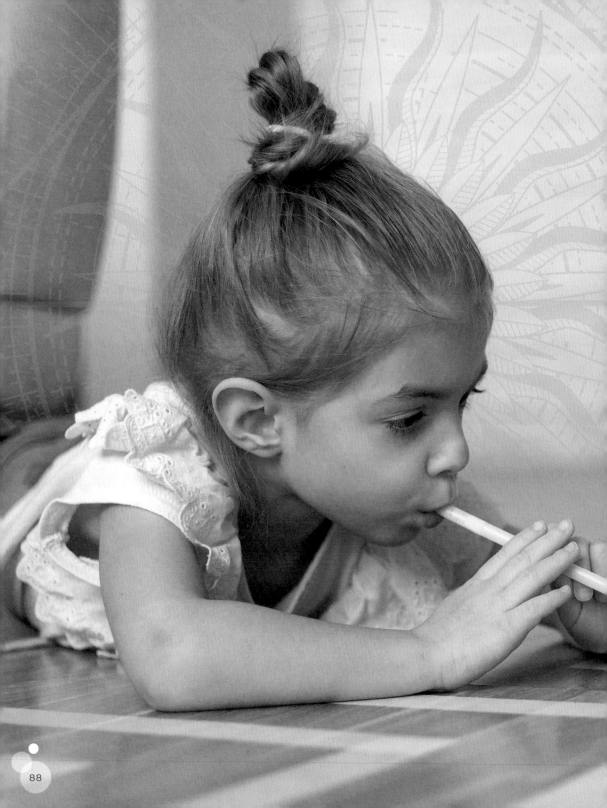

EXERCISE 19
Air soccer: make breathwork into a sporting activity

To make breathwork even more fun, you can turn it into a sporting activity with air soccer. All you'll need is some drinking straws, some lightweight form of ball and more than one child to play the game – or perhaps your child can play against you! They will be getting some breathwork practice without realizing it, strengthening their lungs and taking in lots of oxygen.

How to practise

Ask the children to lie on their bellies on the floor and give each of them a drinking straw. If there are just two children they can lie facing each other about a half a metre apart. If you have many kids, ask them to form a circle facing each other. Create a small goal in front of each child perhaps with small beanbags or some pebbles.

Place a cotton ball or something like a ping pong ball on the floor in between the kids and tell them to try and score a goal by just blowing through their straws and not touching the ball. You'll probably end up with a floor covered in saliva so this is not a game to play on your best rug!

If you want to make it competitive, the winner can be the first child to score a goal, or to score a certain number of goals. If a competitive adult sports fan is also involved, you'll probably end up with some sort of league table and a cup final happening live on your kitchen floor!

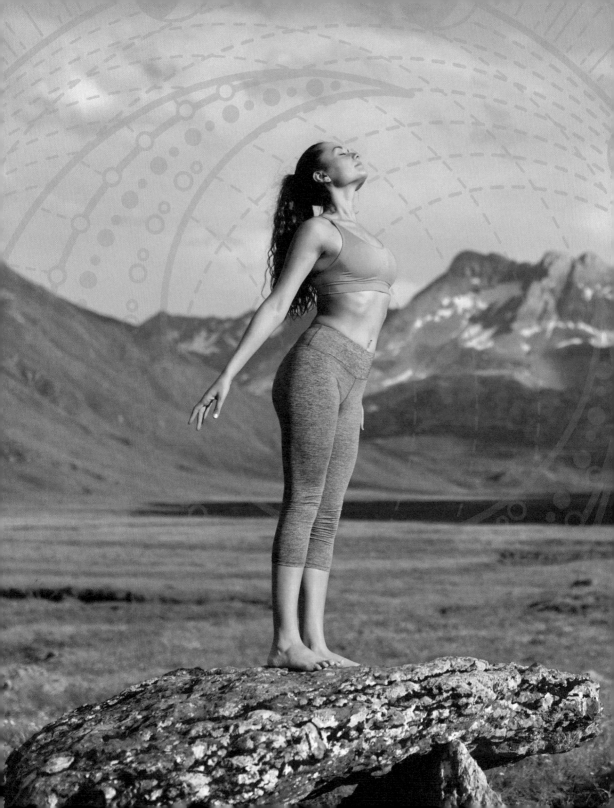

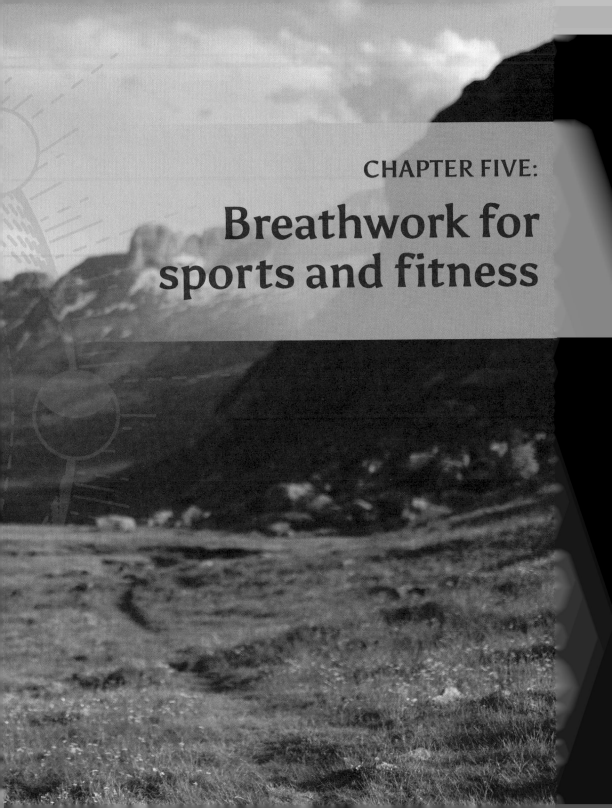

CHAPTER FIVE:

Breathwork for sports and fitness

Turn your body into a more efficient machine

Although breathwork is often associated with serene and peaceful things like meditation and yoga, it is also used by most professional athletes as part of their training routine. The rapid absorption of oxygen into the blood, plus the removal of waste gases, is absolutely essential when it comes to making the body more efficient.

In some high-tech training gyms you'll even see athletes hooked up to breathing tubes while they are on a treadmill or static exercise bike, so that a medical team can then analyze how efficient their breathing is. Most of us won't need this level of high-tech training for our own sporting activities but there are still some easy breathwork exercises that will help improve your breathing efficiency even if the most sport you do is a weekly game of Badminton.

Try out some of the following exercises and you should notice an improvement in your breathing while taking part in a sporting activity, or even when just running up and down stairs in your house or office.

EXERCISE 20
Rapid fire breathing: to help prime your body for sporting activity

This breathwork exercise is often performed by athletes before they start their warm-up exercises. It's a rapid breathing technique that boosts your energy levels and makes you feel very alert. As a fairly intensive exercise it may not be suitable for those with breathing problems or for those who are pregnant.

How to practise

For this exercise you can either be standing up or in a seated position, but in both cases your back should be straight and your neck and head also straight. Your shoulders should be relaxed and down as well as slightly back.

Then, using just your nose, inhale rapidly for one second then exhale rapidly for another one second. The breaths shouldn't be deep diaphragmatic ones but fairly short chest breaths that can be repeated in quick succession.

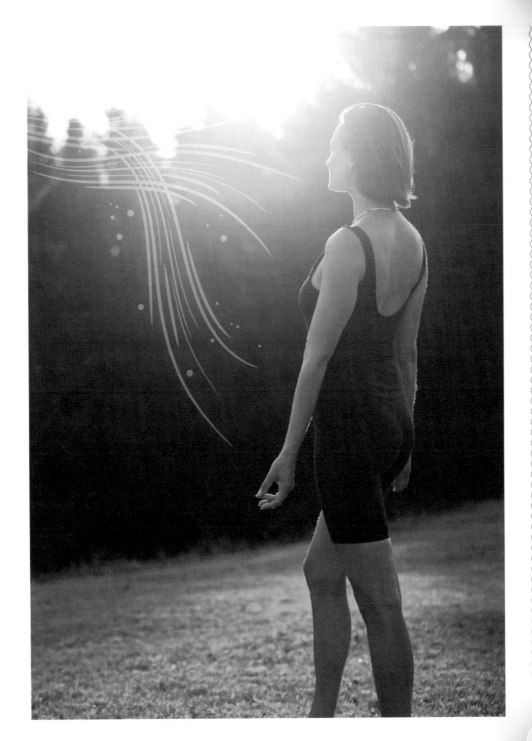

Continue breathing like this for just a couple of minutes. You may start to feel a little light-headed but if this isn't too much you can work through it. If you begin to feel really dizzy just stop for a few minutes and take slow, deep breaths.

After this exercise you should feel really awake and full of energy, ready to start your sporting activity.

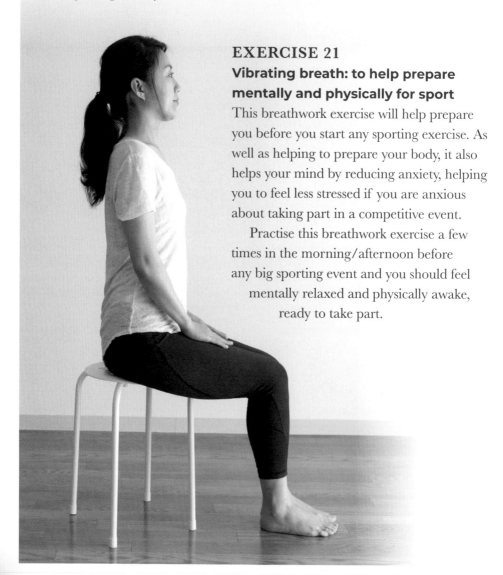

EXERCISE 21
Vibrating breath: to help prepare mentally and physically for sport

This breathwork exercise will help prepare you before you start any sporting exercise. As well as helping to prepare your body, it also helps your mind by reducing anxiety, helping you to feel less stressed if you are anxious about taking part in a competitive event.

Practise this breathwork exercise a few times in the morning/afternoon before any big sporting event and you should feel mentally relaxed and physically awake, ready to take part.

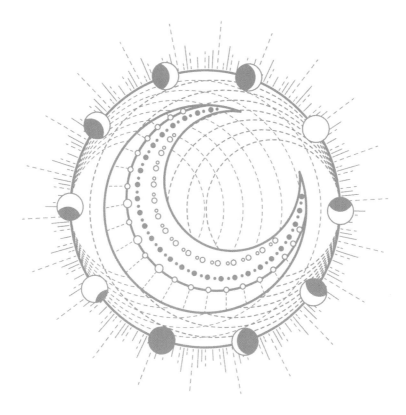

How to practise

Sit in an upright position, either cross-legged on the floor or in a chair. Keep your back straight, your head up and your shoulders relaxed and down.

With your lips closed, breathe in slowly through your nose and fill your lungs. Then exhale slowly through your closed lips, so that they vibrate and your breath makes a humming sound like a bee.

Enjoy the feeling of the vibration and let your cheeks vibrate as well as your lips. Feel the buzzing sensation throughout your whole body and make the buzzing sound as loud as you want.

Continue breathing like this for around five minutes, or for as long as you want, perhaps just stopping for short breaks of normal breathing in between sets of buzzing breathing.

EXERCISE 22
Roaring lion's breath:
to release tension and prepare you for active sport

This exercise is great for releasing tension, particularly in your face and upper body. Mentally, it makes you feel like a roaring lion, ready to take on any sporting opponent.

How to practise

On a yoga mat or soft floor, get into a cross-legged seating position or kneel if you prefer.

Then, either press the palms of your hands onto your knees or, if you are more flexible, place the palms of your hands on the floor in front of you and spread out your fingers. Imagine that you are a lion in its seated position.

Then inhale deeply through your nose, keeping your eyes wide open and looking forward. At the same time open your mouth wide and stick out your tongue. Make your tongue as long as possible and tip it down towards your chin.

Then contract the muscles at the front of your throat and exhale through your mouth making a long 'haaa' sound. While you are breathing out, look up with your open eyes, as if focusing on a space between your eyebrows or focus on the tip of your nose.

You should feel like a wild lion, making as much noise as you want.

Repeat the breath in sets of five or 10 at a time, perhaps with three sets in total.

After you should feel fit and aware, like a lion on the hunt for sporting victory!

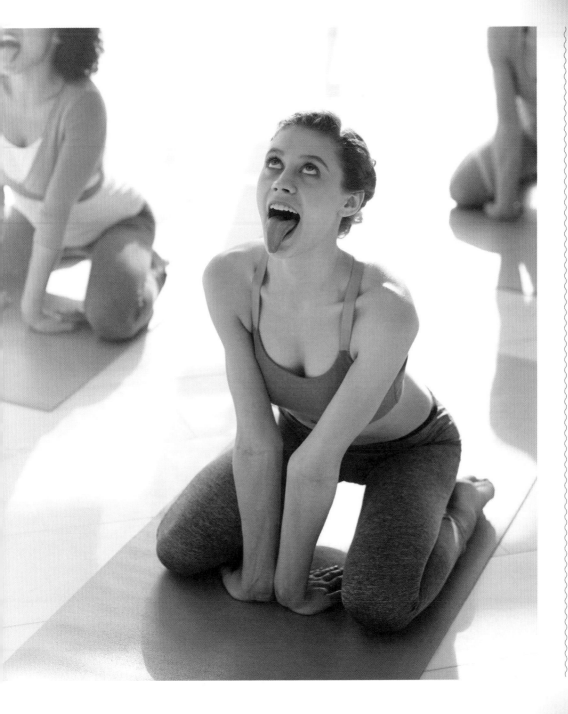

EXERCISE 23
Recovery breathing: to help your body recover after sporting activity

As well as helping you to prepare for sporting activity, breathwork can also help you to recover after an intensive period of exercise. This simple technique will help your body to relax and get back to normal once your intensive exercise has finished.

How to practise

Lie on your back with your feet facing a wall or a chair. Then raise your legs and bend your knees, so that your lower legs are at 90 degrees to your upper legs. You can then either support your feet against the wall or rest your lower legs and feet on the seat of a chair.

Spread your arms slightly apart down either side of your body and make sure your lower back is in a comfortable position, perhaps with a small pillow under it if needed.

Spend a few seconds to relax your body as much as possible then begin the breathwork.

Start by taking a slow, deep breath in through your nose and feel as your lower back pushes into the floor. Make a count of five in your head as you slowly breathe in and fill your lungs.

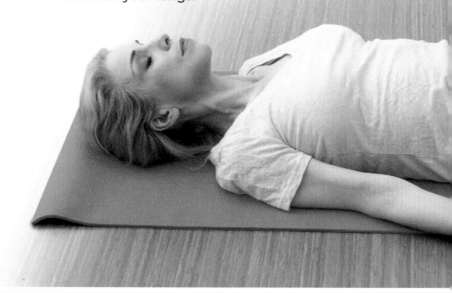

Then, hold the breath in for another count of five, noticing how your lower back and shoulders are pressed against the floor.

Finally, exhale through your nose for another count of five and notice how your lower back lifts a little.

Carry on breathing like this for around five minutes, until you feel your body has totally relaxed after exercise and that any soreness in your legs or arms or any other part of your body created during the exercise has receded, as your muscles recover their normal chemical balance and oxygen levels.

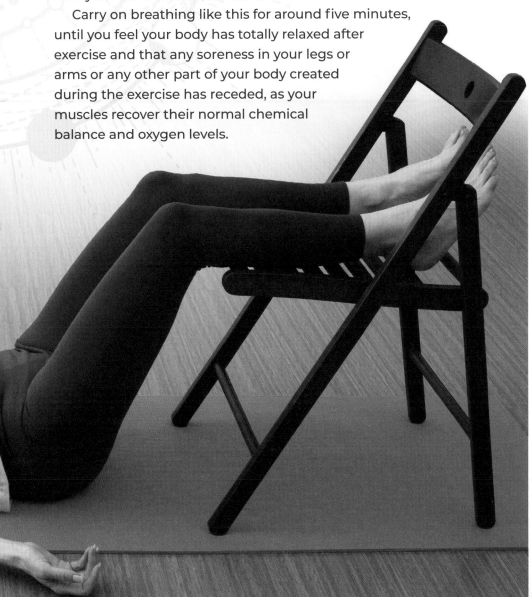

CHAPTER SIX

Breathwork to help you sleep

Focusing your mind away from stress and anxiety

When I told the mother of a friend of mine that I was writing a book on breathwork, I was surprised that she told me she has her own breathwork technique which she uses if she is finding it hard to sleep at night. So, the first of the exercises below is her own, simple breathing exercise; if it works for her then hopefully it might help you as well, if you have sleeping problems.

I will also include some other, well-known breathing techniques for helping you relax and sleep at night.

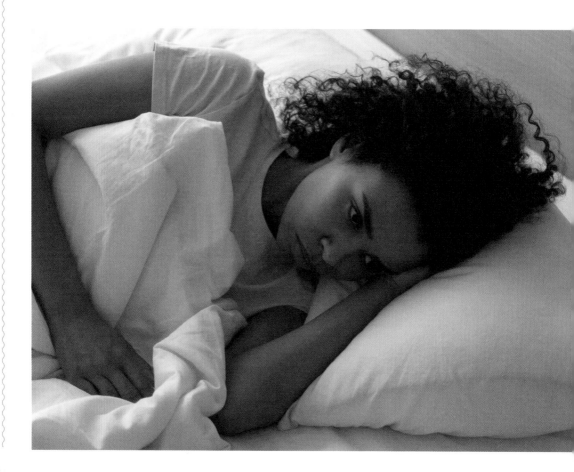

EXERCISE 24
Simple breath focus: a relaxing and easy technique to start with

This is the breathwork technique practised by the mother of a friend of mine, called Joan. Back in the 1970s, with two small kids to look after, Joan was a keen practitioner of that trendy, 'new' hippy fad called yoga, so she became aware of the importance of breathing alongside the yoga asanas (postures).

Over time she developed her own, simple breathwork technique which she practices when she is in bed at night but is having problems getting off to sleep. So, this is a well-proven technique and is based on some other well-known breathwork techniques.

How to practise

Practise this technique when you are lying in bed, trying to relax and get off to sleep, or perhaps do it just before you go to bed and when you are sitting up in a chair.

Start by taking a deep breath in through your nose, counting slowly to three in your head as you do so. Fill your lungs up and notice your chest rising.

Then, hold your breath in for another count of three, feeling how full your lungs are.

Finally breathe out slowly and completely through your nose, during another count of three in your head. Enjoy the experience of emptying your lungs of all those waste gases.

You can do this as many times as you want, but Joan says that she usually only does about five breaths like this, which she finds relaxes her and helps to send her off to sleep.

One of the main reasons that exercises like this work is because you are mentally concentrating on your breath, which takes your mind off other stressful things and therefore helps you to relax. That's why breathing exercises are often used as the way into meditation practice, helping to focus the mind away from other thoughts.

EXERCISE 25

Body scan breathing: to feel your whole body relax, ready for sleep

As with the mantra technique, body scanning is often used as a meditation technique, where you focus on your body to take your mind off other things. Combining this with thinking about your breath and some simple breathwork exercises is also a great way to relax before bed.

You can also use this technique to focus on parts of your body that may be in pain, removing tension and stress plus sending positive healing energy.

How to practise

Lie down on your bed, or on something like a comfortable yoga mat, and breathe normally through your nose for a minute or so, focusing on your breath, sensing your chest moving and your lungs filling and emptying.

Feel how your body is being supported by the bed or mat, release all your tension into the bed so that your body is totally relaxed. At the same time, continue to focus on your breath, with slow and steady inhalations and exhalations.

Now begin to mentally scan your body, concentrating on individual parts. Start with your head: how does it feel, is it totally relaxed or does it feel tense? Then slowly move down to focusing on your shoulders, arms, chest and the rest of your body in turn, ending up with your toes. Spend 10 or 20 seconds focusing on each part of your body then move on to the next. If the muscles in the parts you are focusing on seem tense, aim to relax them by feeling them being fully supported by the bed. Be aware of your breathing throughout, taking slow, regular breaths.

Once you have scanned your whole body like this, concentrate fully on your slow breathing and start repeating a mantra in your head every time you exhale. This could be something with a few words like 'feel relaxed' or just a single word like 'sleep'. Continue like this for perhaps another five minutes or so, or until you really feel sleepy. You may just drop off to sleep anyway, which would be perfect.

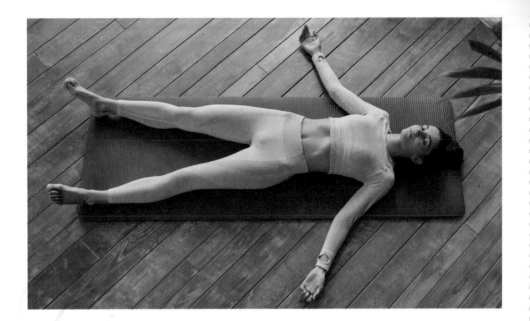

In meditation, body scanning like this can take 30 minutes or so, but you might find 10 or 15 minutes is enough when combined with a focus on breathing like this. You don't need to save this form of breathwork for nighttime, it can be good at other times of day as well, perhaps to reduce stress in the middle of a busy day, before carrying on refreshed and relaxed.

EXERCISE 26
Closed breath breathing: to help set a relaxed breathing rhythm before sleep

When we are very stressed, our breathing rhythm is usually broken as well, in the worst cases leading to hyperventilation. As part of relaxing and getting ready for sleep, we need to recover a more natural breathing pattern and focus away from the stresses in our lives.

Although it might seem a little extreme, this exercise can help you to reset a more normal breathing state.

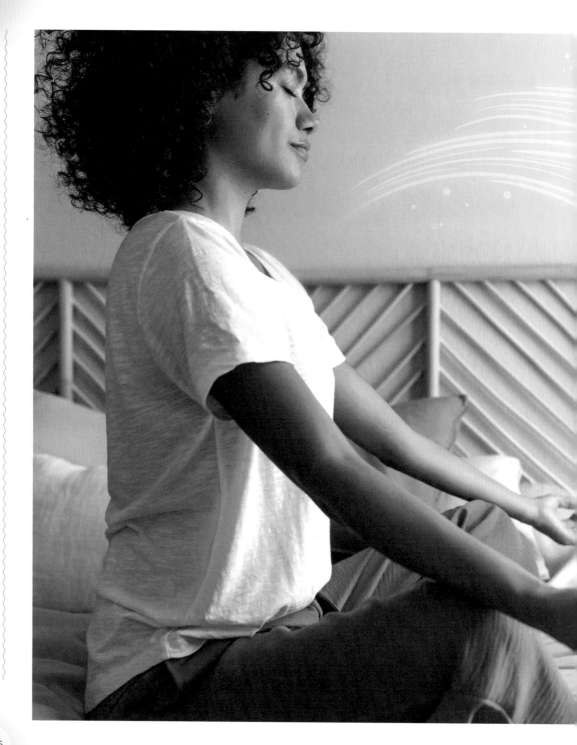

How to practise

Sit in a comfortable position, perhaps propped up with cushions in your bed, but make sure your back is straight and your shoulders are down and relaxed.

Close your mouth gently and breathe normally through your nose for a minute or so.

Then take a deep breath in and out through your nose and pinch your nose closed with your thumb and forefinger once your lungs are empty. Keep your mouth closed as well and stay like this, with empty lungs, until you feel that you really need to take another breath in. The time for this period of keeping your lungs empty will vary between different people and could be anything from 10 seconds to 30 seconds and it's better to do this for a shorter period of time when you first start practising this exercise, then build up to a longer time.

Finally, with your mouth still closed, take a deep breath in and out through your nose again.

Relax for a few seconds and see how you feel. You can repeat this exercise up to five times, then stop for a period of normal breathing. Do a few more sets of five if you feel like it, but you may already be feeling more sleepy and relaxed after just a few breaths like this.

As well as helping you to sleep, this breathwork exercise can also help to calm you down if you are having a panic attack, providing that you have the presence of mind to do breathwork at this time.

EXERCISE 27
Whoosh breathing: make some noise to quieten your mind

It might seem a bit counter-intuitive that breathwork which makes a noise can help quieten and calm you down, but forgetting our inhibitions and not worrying about noise can also be an important part of the de-stressing and relaxing process, along with the actual breathwork benefits. This exercise doesn't make too much noise, just a gentle whooshing sound, so you shouldn't bother the neighbours too much at night!

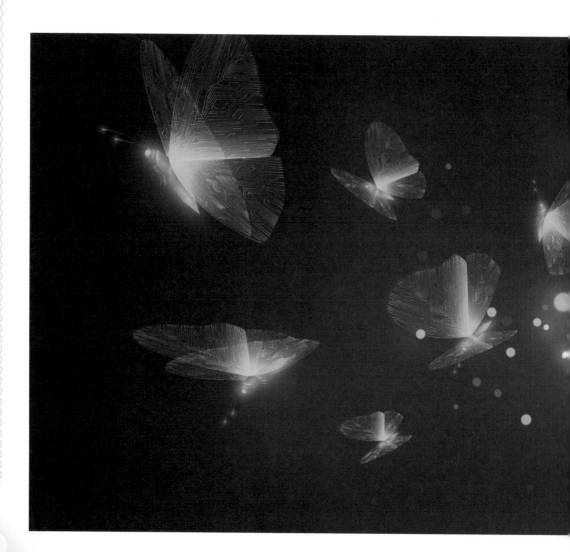

How to practise

Get into a comfortable seated position, possibly in bed, making sure your back is straight and shoulders are relaxed and down. You could also do this exercise when standing if you want, but this might not be quite so relaxing afterwards.

Take a deep breath in through your nose, counting to four in your head as you fill your lungs with air.

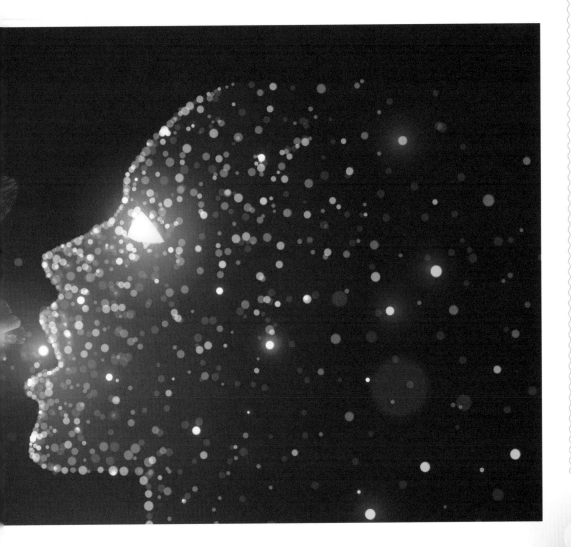

Hold your breath for a count of six, then let your lips part gently and exhale through them so that the air makes a whooshing sound as it exits your mouth. Fully exhale all the air from your lungs like this while counting to six.

Repeat this breath five times, then relax before doing a few more sets of five if you feel like it.

EXERCISE 28
Countdown breathing: count yourself to sleep while focusing on your breathing

We've all heard about counting sheep to help send yourself to sleep and this breathwork technique draws on that idea, combining breathing with counting numbers in your head.

How to practise
Lie down in bed, getting comfortable and preparing yourself for sleep. Feel the mattress and pillow supporting all of your body and relax deeply into them.

Now start to concentrate on your breathing. Carry on breathing in a relaxed, normal way through your nose but start counting with every exhalation, starting with one, two, three... etc. for each exhalation.

Before you begin you can set yourself a target, say counting up to 50, but hopefully you will fall asleep before getting there. If not, once you reach your target start counting back down to one with each exhale.

To elaborate and focus the mind even more, you can make the process more about imagery. Find an image to match the counting. This could be one sheep jumping over a fence for each count, or one green bottle being sat on top of a wall for each count, or perhaps one brick being added to a wall and imagining the wall growing with each brick.

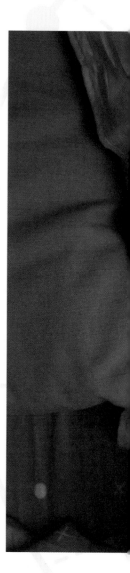

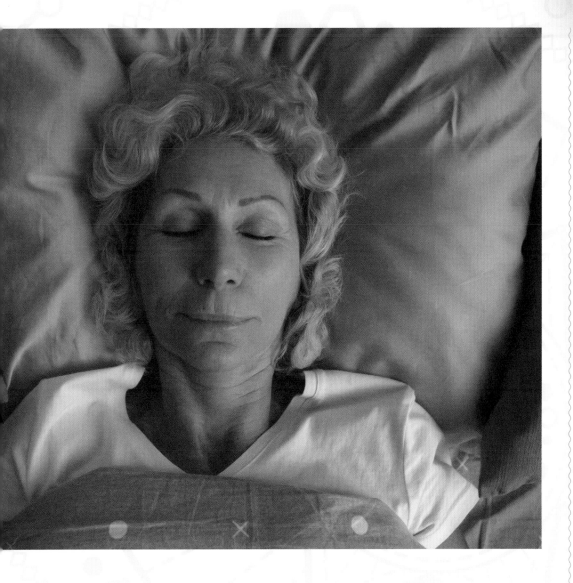

Just find something that works for you, or stick to counting numbers and keep it simple.

The main thing is to link the counting with each exhaled breath, so both your mind and body are focused on the activity, clearing your head from other thoughts and relaxing you into sleep.

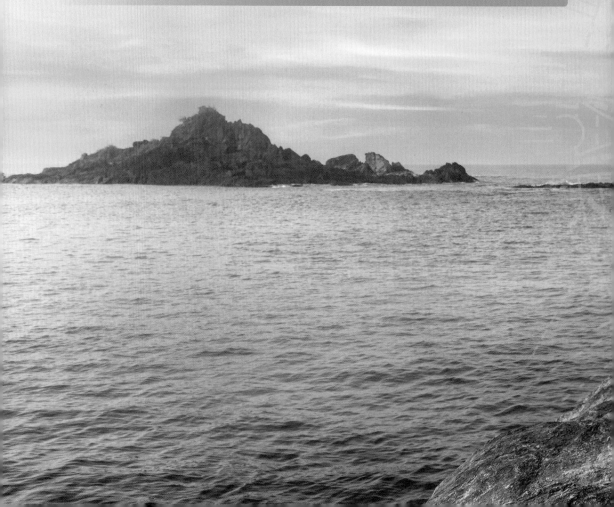

CHAPTER SEVEN:

Breathwork at a more advanced level

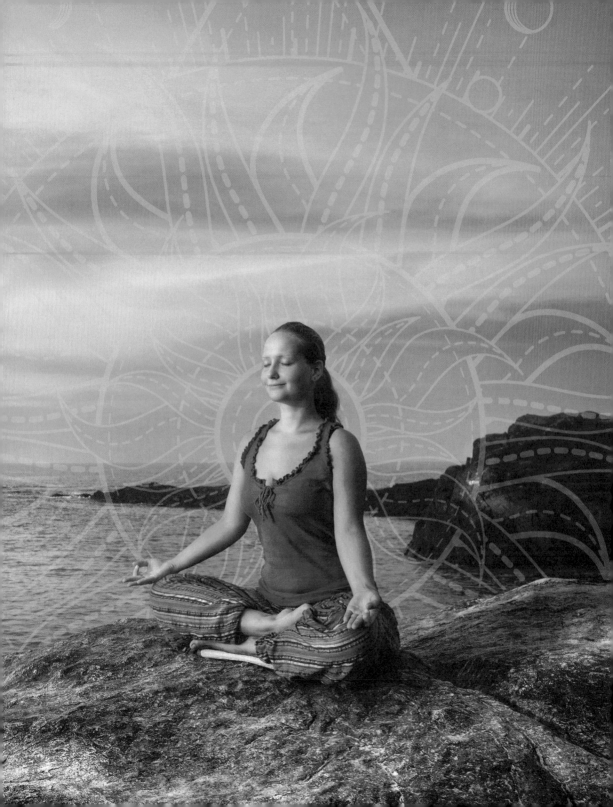

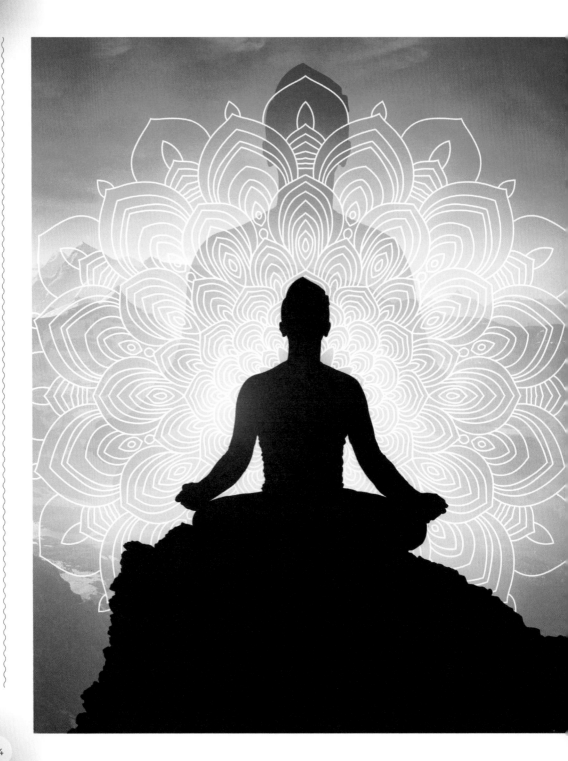

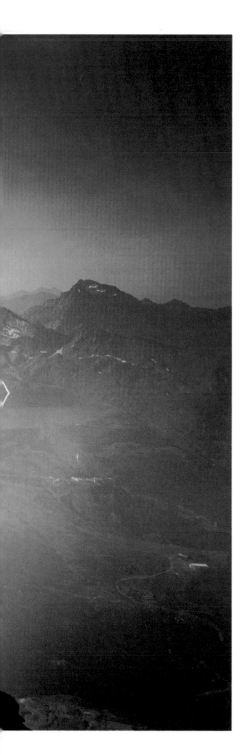

More intensive techniques

Some breathwork exercises are a little more intensive and shouldn't really be tried until you are fully confident in your abilities and have spent time practising many of the simpler exercises.

If you are healthy then none of these exercises should present any problems but if you suffer from conditions such as asthma or other lung diseases, or if you have heart-related problems, then the over-stimulation of more extreme breathwork exercises might not be good.

If you have any concerns, speak to your doctor before undertaking more extreme breathwork exercises.

In addition, it is usually not recommended that anyone who is pregnant undertakes really intensive breathwork exercises. It is very unlikely to cause a problem, but the general shock to the system might make you feel a little dizzy.

It's good to tune into your body's feelings and reactions and never push yourself if a breathwork exercise is making you feel dizzy or nauseous. Just stop and take a break, perhaps lie down for a few minutes until you feel fine again.

I would also recommend finding an expert, such as a fully qualified yoga teacher, who can show you the ropes when it comes to more intensive breathwork exercises, plus offer support.

EXERCISE 29

Kapalabhati breathing or shining face breathing: a natural face-lift!

One of the more common breathing techniques used in yoga practice, Kapalabhati breathing, is fairly intensive and is said to make your face and forehead more shiny and refreshed. It also helps to flush out your respiratory system and can even help stimulate your digestive system.

The main feeling people get when practising Kapalabhati is exhilaration, as your blood oxygen levels rise fairly quickly.

If you are not used to breathwork exercises, then Kapalabhati breathing can make you feel a little dizzy so just stop and relax if this happens, with slow, deep breathing.

How to practise

Put yourself into a comfortable seated position, either on a chair or in a cross-legged yoga posture, and keep your back straight and upright. Start by breathing in gently and fully, through your nose and with your

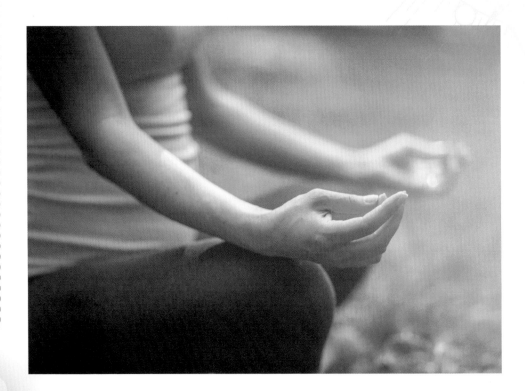

mouth closed, using your diaphragm and abdominal muscles, feeling your chest expand.

Then, with your mouth remaining closed, make a quick and forceful exhalation of breath through your nose. Use your diaphragm and abdominal muscles to force the air out quickly. This quick exhalation through your nose should make quite a sound and a room full of people practicing Kapalabhati breathing often sounds like a load of steam trains setting off from a station!

Once you have mastered the technique you need to do these breaths quickly one after the other in a number of sets. I usually do 30 Kapalabhati breaths in one set, then relax for a minute or so, before doing another set of 30. I usually do three sets of 30 Kapalabhati breaths as part of a yoga session. If you are new to Kapalabhati breathing, you might want to reduce the number of breaths in one set, perhaps down to 10 instead of 30, plus do fewer sets. Just see how your body reacts and whether it makes you feel dizzy or not.

The main thing to be aware of is that your inhalation should feel passive and easy, but your exhalation should feel forced and quick.

I find that students are usually glowing and mentally buzzing after a Kapalabhati breathing session and I usually move onto more intensive yoga asanas (postures) afterwards.

EXERCISE 30
Bellows breathing or Bhastrika: for an even shinier face!

Often seen as the next step up from Kapalabhati breathing, Bhastrika or bellows breathing involves both the forceful and quick exhalation and inhalation of air. It can give you even more of a 'buzz' than Kapalabhati breathing but there's also a slightly greater risk of feeling dizzy if you overdo it.

As with Kapalabhati, this exercise is not recommended if you are pregnant or have any lung or heart problems as it is intensive and can be a bit of a shock to the system if you are not used to it.

How to practise

Again, put yourself into a comfortable seated position, either on a chair or in a cross-legged yoga posture, and keep your back straight and upright. Your mouth should remain shut throughout this exercise, with all the breathing done through your nose.

Start by breathing in fully, forcefully and quickly through your nose, using your diaphragm and abdominal muscles to suck in the air. Feel your lungs expand fully.

Then, with your mouth still remaining closed, make a quick and forceful exhalation of breath through your nose. Use your diaphragm and abdominal muscles to force the air out quickly.

As with Kapalabhati, this quick inhalation and exhalation should make a lot of noise, and can be even more exhilarating when practised with loads of other people at the same time, such as in a yoga class.

Don't worry if you throw out mucus through your nose while doing this exercise; that's quite natural, even if it might not look so good to others around you!

As with Kapalabhati, these breaths should be done in quick succession and in small sets, but you may want to do fewer breaths in each set. Between 10 and 15 breaths should be enough for each set. Then relax for a minute before starting the next set. Three sets may be enough but just see how you feel.

If you feel dizzy during or after this breathing exercise, just lie down for a few minutes, then get up slowly. Or, if it's not so bad, just stay in your seated position as any dizziness usually goes in a few seconds.

I usually only practise this breathing exercise with my more advanced yoga students, mainly because I think they will benefit from it more and not because of any fears of it causing any problems such as dizziness.

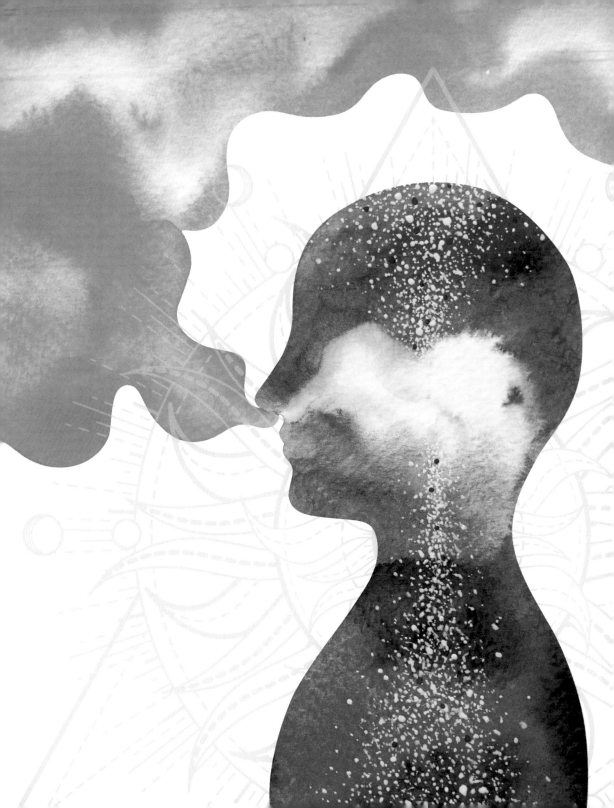

EXERCISE 31

Held-breath breathing: to strengthen lungs and refresh the mind

This exercise also builds on Kapalabhati but this time with a period of holding in your breath. This allows an even greater exchange of gases in your lungs, with more oxygen going into your bloodstream and more carbon dioxide being expelled. It can also help to increase your lung capacity and strength, as well as helping to force out excess phlegm.

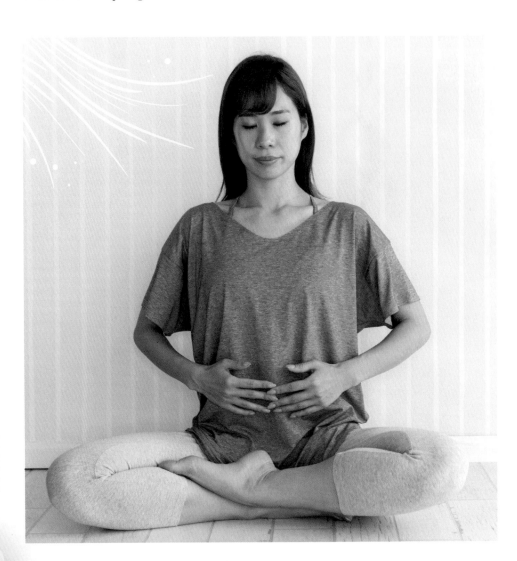

Again it is not recommended for people with chest or heart problems, or for those who are pregnant, due to its intensity more than anything else.

How to practise

Get yourself into a comfortable seated position, either on a chair or in a cross-legged yoga posture, and keep your back straight and upright. Your mouth should remain shut throughout this exercise, with all the breathing done through your nose.

Start by breathing in fully, forcefully and quickly through your nose, using your diaphragm and abdominal muscles to suck in the air. Feel your lungs expand fully.

Then, with your mouth still remaining closed, make a quick and forceful exhalation of breath through your nose. Use your diaphragm and abdominal muscles to force the air out quickly.

Do nine breaths like this in quick succession then, after the tenth inhalation, hold all the air in your lungs for a count of five to 10 (or for as long as feels comfortable), then exhale all the air slowly back through your nose. Fully empty your lungs in a slow and gradual way.

Then rest for a while taking normal breaths before starting the process again. Aim to do at least three sets of this exercise if you can, but monitor your body throughout and only do what feels comfortable for you.

If you feel dizzy during or after this breathing exercise, just lie down for a few minutes. Or, just stay in your seated position as any dizziness usually goes in a few seconds.

This is probably one of the most advanced breathing exercises as the quick breathing in and out, combined with holding in the air for a period of time, gives your body a massive oxygen boost, at a time when you're stationary and not doing any exercise to immediately use up the oxygen. Your body will eventually store all the excess oxygen as energy, so you should feel an energy boost for quite a while afterwards.

EXERCISE 32

Victorious breath or ujjayi breathing: to calm your mind and release tension

This breathwork technique is often used as part of a mindfulness session as it concentrates your focus on your breathing which in turn calms all your other thoughts and clears the mind. Yogis refer to this type of breathwork as *ujjayi* pranayama or breathing. It is seen as a type of breathwork that can mentally free you from bondage and bring you victory, perhaps helping you to win out against the stresses and strains of your daily life.

It is also thought to help improve your mood and make you feel happier, as well as relieving anxiety and even helping to increase and regulate body temperature. It has even been used to help relieve anxiety in patients with cancer, sometimes having a positive effect on some symptoms as well.

It can also help to relieve insomnia since it has a profoundly relaxing effect and can help with sleep when carried out before bedtime. It can also reduce blood pressure and slow down the heart rate.

How to practise

Sit in a position that's comfortable for you, ideally in a cross-legged yoga pose with your hands on your knees, palms facing upwards. Or, if you prefer, you can just sit upright in a chair. In all cases, sit with your back straight and your shoulders relaxed, plus with your eyes closed.

Start by focusing on your breath; sense the air coming in through your nose and into your lungs and allow your breathing to become calm and rhythmic.

Continue breathing normally like this but start to imagine that the air is being drawn in and out through the throat and not through the nose. Imagine that inhalation and exhalation is taking place through a hole in your throat.

Now try and tighten your throat so that a soft snoring sound, like a sleeping baby, is heard as you breathe in and out. You may find that your abdomen contracts at the same time.

With your throat constricted like this, breathe in slowly until your chest is full, then hold your breath for a count of five, then breathe out slowly.

Throughout, your face and nose should be as relaxed as possible, with all the focus on your constricted throat.

Repeat this breathing for a set of 10 to 15 breaths, then relax a little, before doing more sets, perhaps three to five sets in total. You can do this several times a day to get the maximum benefit.

Final thoughts

I hope you enjoy practising the breathwork techniques covered in the book and that you find them helpful to both your physical and mental health. Writing the book has made me focus even more on my own breathwork practice, trying a wider variety of techniques than I had before, as well as teaching these to my yoga and mindfulness students.

I have also found that my daily nasal cleansing practice has been very effective. I wash the inside of my nose and nasal cavity every morning and this sets me up for the day, both physically and mentally. It has also made breathwork easier, since I was often a little congested before, but regular nasal cleansing has done away with this. I suspect that regular cleaning like this, with a mild saline solution, will also help to reduce the impact of cold bugs and flu viruses and I haven't had a cold since upping my nose cleaning to a daily rather than a once-a-week practice.

With regular breathwork practice I feel much fitter when it comes to exercise such as hiking and cycling. It's interesting to see that professional sports coaches are now recognizing the importance of breathwork as part of the training routine for athletes, even going so far as to monitor athletes' breathing efficiency by putting them on a treadmill and making them breathe through a mask that's connected to high-tech monitoring equipment.

Most of us won't need to go to that extreme to feel the benefits of regular breathwork and I wish you all the best with your own practice.

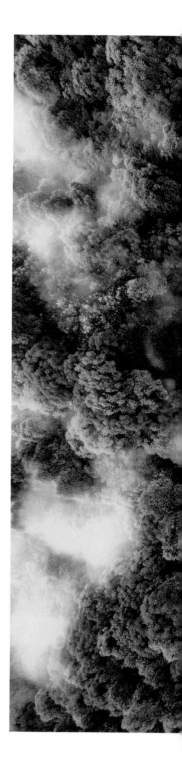

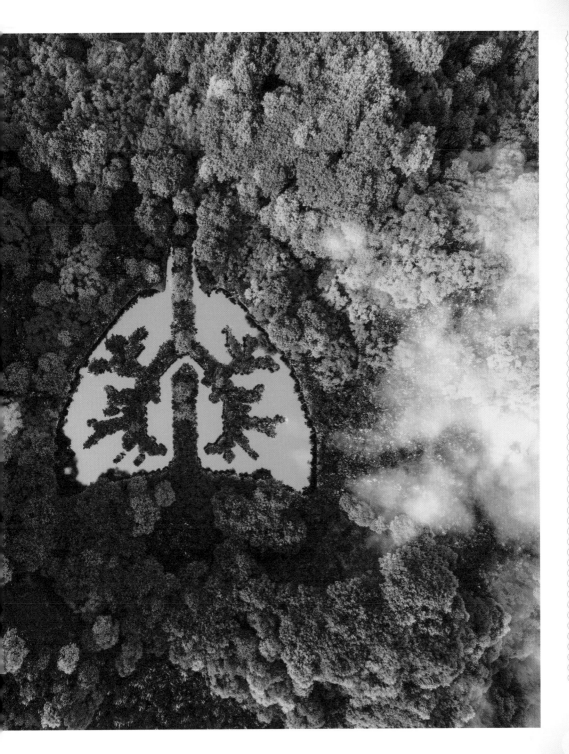

About the author

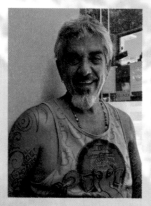

Konstantinos Tselios is a Greek-born mindfulness and senior yoga teacher, based in both London and on the Greek island of Crete. He is also a magazine journalist and book author, writing about yoga and alternative health and spirituality in a series of features published in *Kindred Spirit* and *Prediction* magazines in the UK, as well as writing a book on Ayurveda, from the same publishers as this book.

He has travelled widely, with many trips to India over the past 20 years, gaining some of his yoga teaching qualifications there. He is also a qualified mindfulness teacher, carrying out classes in person as well as online.

In 2014, Kostas was diagnosed with Stage 4 bowel cancer, requiring an emergency operation, followed up by chemotherapy. This made him even more interested in complementary medicines and techniques such as breathwork, which he used to help rebuild his strength and boost his recovery. He also found that breathwork and meditation helped with his state of mind and mental health when battling cancer.

This advice is now something he passes on to students, including breathwork techniques which he teaches as part of his yoga instruction and mindfulness coaching.

Konstantinos can be contacted by email at: costastselios@yahoo.com

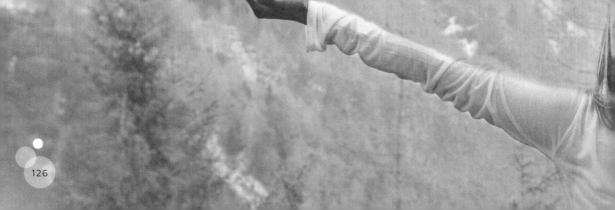

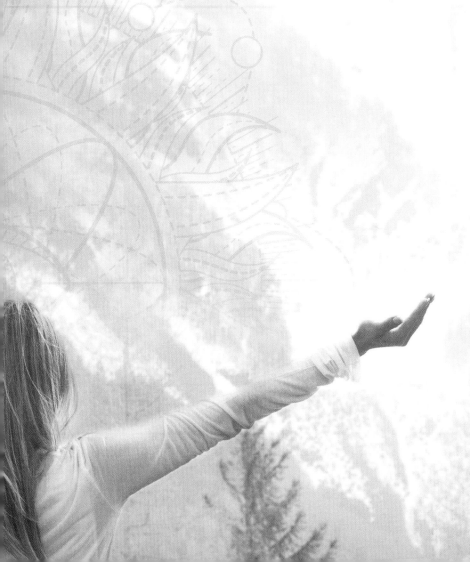

Acknowledgements

The author would like to thank those who helped with this book, including
Steve Rowe for his editing work, Joan Rowe for her copy-checking skills, plus
Tania O'Donnell for commissioning him to write it and the team at Arcturus for
publishing it. He also wants to thank the many people and organizations that have
helped him with his own health issues over the years, and the many teachers and
gurus who have guided him on his spiritual path.

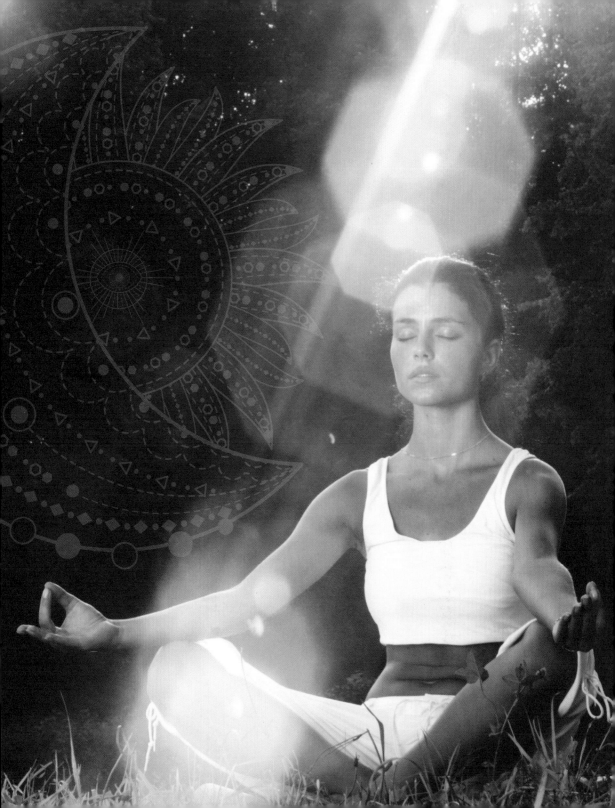